✳ the hugely better slimming plan

essentials

✳ the hugely better slimming plan

essentials

carolyn humphries

foulsham

LONDON • NEW YORK • TORONTO • SYDNEY

foulsham

The Publishing House, Bennetts Close, Cippenham,
Slough, Berkshire, SL1 5AP, England

ISBN 0-572-02842-3

Neither the editors of W. Foulsham & Co. Ltd nor the author nor the publisher take
responsibility for any possible consequences from any treatment, procedure, test,
exercise, action or application of medication or preparation by any person reading
or following the information in this book. The publication of this book does not
constitute the practice of medicine, and this book does not attempt to replace any
diet or instructions from your doctor. The author and publisher advise the reader
to check with a doctor before administering any medication or undertaking any
course of treatment or exercise.

Printed in Great Britain by Cox & Wyman Ltd, Reading, Berkshire

Contents

Introduction 7

The Pros and Cons of Different Diets 11

Healthy Eating for Life 24

Wise Ways to Weight Reduction 32

Lifestyle Quiz 40

Using the Diet Plan 55

Your 28-day Diet Plan 65

Special Occasions 95

Maintaining the New You 100

Everyday Diet Plan Recipes 102

Special-occasion Diet Plan Recipes 164

Index 189

Introduction

It's here at last! A diet for those of us who have no will-power, and need a bar of chocolate, a gin and tonic, a packet of nibbles or other comfort foods or drinks to keep body and soul together. It's not faddy, it's not a crash plan – this is a complete package that will allow you your treats and won't leave you with hunger pangs. What's more, it offers you a healthy, well-balanced diet to make you a fitter, more vital person. Most important, of course, it will help you lose weight.

No one needs to be told that crash diets don't work – we all know not only that they are bad for us but also that they don't work because the weight just goes back on as soon as we stop following them. This diet plan is different: it's about a gradual, effortless weight loss, so if you use the whole package from the beginning, you can keep up the regime for as long as it takes for you to reach and maintain your target weight.

The diet is made up of 28 complete meal plans – that's four weeks'-worth – and each one is made up of three delicious meals, plus snacks and treats! If you want to lose a few pounds quickly, or if you want to kick-start your diet, then you can follow the diet without any of the snacks, then introduce the full snacks-allowed regime after a couple of weeks.

Because it's a healthy eating plan, you can follow it for as long as you like. In fact, using this plan to introduce you to a healthy eating habit is one of the most important factors towards success in your diet.

So why should this diet be any more successful than any other? There are lots of reasons.

- It's based on sound nutritional advice: this is a healthy, balanced diet.
- It's easy to follow because all the thinking is done for you; there are no points or calories to calculate or worry about.
- You can use either ready-made or home-made dishes to suit your lifestyle.
- It gives you the low-down on all the diets you've tried – and probably some that you haven't – with their advantages and disadvantages, so you understand where you may have gone wrong in the past.
- It's designed especially with everyone's strengths and weaknesses in mind.

So how does it work?

Each one of us knows where we fall down when we are trying to lose weight: that mid-morning snack, that extra helping of pud, that glass of wine – and we try to pretend it doesn't matter! But once you've answered the fun quiz on pages 40–45, you won't be able to kid yourself any more. You'll know exactly what sort of eater you are, how to work with your strengths – and how to overcome your weaknesses.

This little book will tell you everything you need to know about dieting and making it work for you. Read on and you'll find a tasty, nutritious diet that includes plenty of convenience foods as well as home-cooked meals, snacks and treats. It'll tell you what to eat when you go out and there are even some delicious special recipes for when you're entertaining at home. And with advice on a long-term eating plan, you'll be able to maintain your healthy eating – and your new trimmer figure – with ease.

How to Use This Book

The first thing you need to know is how much weight you want to lose. Remember, being underweight is no better than being overweight, and neither is good for your health – so look at the chart on page 28 and work out what your correct weight range should be.

It is also important that you understand how and why this diet will work. Chapters 1 and 2, The Pros and Cons of Different Diets and Healthy Eating for Life, give you all the information you need to understand what your body really needs to stay fit and how to achieve a well-balanced diet.

Next, fill in the quiz starting on page 40. This is designed to find out more about your individual likes and dislikes, your habits and your weaknesses. It will also show what sort of diet will suit you and how you can eat more healthily and lose weight more effectively.

A positive attitude and motivation to succeed are crucial if you are to achieve your dieting goals. Chapter 3, Wise Ways to Weight Reduction, will show you how to increase your chances of success by getting yourself in the right frame of mind.

Now you're ready to begin the diet. So start today – and enjoy it!

Chapter 1
The Pros and Cons of Different Diets

Most of us have tried a variety of diets – and sadly, the statistics prove that most of them don't work, although it's not always clear why. I've studied all the different kinds of diets that are available, and researched the principles on which they are based, according to their creators. I've looked at what's good and not so good about them, and why, for the most part, they are unlikely to work as a long-term solution to your weight problem.

Why do you need to know all this?

Because it will demonstrate to you that the only way to lose weight and maintain a healthy weight is to follow a perfectly balanced, calorie-controlled diet. To stay healthy, you must have all the nutrients your body needs to thrive. To stick to any diet, you need to eat food you enjoy – and to be able to indulge in some of life's little pleasures as well.

With the eating plan in this book, you can control your calorie intake for just as long as you need to lose weight, by which time you should be so used to enjoying your healthier diet, you won't need to stay strictly on the plan any more.

Body toning diets

These suggest a regime based on a very low-fat diet, combined with lots of exercise to reduce weight and tone particular parts of the body. The 'hip and thigh' diet is a good example.

Pros
There is no calorie counting. Vegetables are encouraged on a three-meals-a-day plan and you are allowed snacks if you rearrange the meals to include them. Exercise is an important part of the regime.

Cons
The fat intake is lower than dietetically recommended (see Low-fat Diets, on page 19). The hips and thighs are the fattiest areas of most women so there is nothing magical about weight loss in these areas – they are likely to be the parts to reduce on any reducing diet.

Effectiveness
You will lose weight initially but it won't last long-term unless you stick to the plan and the exercising ... unlikely for most dieters. The fat content is too low for a permanent diet.

Calorie-counted diets

These are very common and very popular. The basic idea is quite simple and perfectly sound: if you eat fewer calories than you burn, you will lose weight.

Pros

Diet sheets are worked out for you, down to the last stick of celery.

Cons

Meals are often small and as they are extremely low in calories – often excessively so – you are likely to feel hungry and cheat. There is little room for flexibility for different lifestyles. Most favourite foods are forbidden.

Effectiveness

When you eat normally again, the weight you have lost – and more – will pile back on.

Detox diets

The body is cleansed by fasting on fruit and/or vegetable juices and water, to remove toxins and help the body to rejuvenate and heal itself. Weight loss will be fast because of the very low calorie intake.

Pros
These diets are easy to follow as there is little choice. They work on a psychological level too – you'll feel good about yourself for what you are doing to your body.

Cons
It is impossible to incorporate this diet into a normal daily routine. The lack of complex carbohydrates and protein will leave you weak and light-headed and your metabolism will slow as you have so few calories to burn. Also, detox diets must be followed for no more than five days at a time.

Effectiveness
This type of diet should be regarded as a quick detox programme, not a long-term diet. It will cause initial weight loss but this loss won't be sustained once you start eating again.

'Exchange' plans

Foods are separated into categories and those within the same group may be exchanged to add variety. Portions are regulated so, for instance, lunch = 2 starch, 1 milk, 1 protein, 1 fruit.

Pros

The plans are nutritionally balanced. You can eat what you fancy within the given framework so this diet will suit different lifestyles. It may be used long-term.

Cons

Weight loss is slow so it's easy to lose heart. It's a chore checking what you're allowed at each meal. You may bore your friends if you try to follow it when you're eating out.

Effectiveness

It can work if you are prepared to persevere but it's so laborious, most people don't.

Fad diets

These include diets such as the 'cabbage soup' diet. You eat an enormous quantity of the fad food, which is claimed to help reduce your weight as part of a bizarre eating plan.

Pros

The diet is rigidly planned so you don't have to work out what to eat.

Cons

Dieting like this is very monotonous and can make you feel nauseous, full of wind or even light-headed. The diets also lack a sensible balance of nutrients and must not be used for more than 10 days maximum, often less.

Effectiveness

You will lose weight while on the diet but it won't last once you start to eat normally again. It doesn't encourage good, long-term eating habits.

Food-combining diets

The best-known of this group is the Hay diet. The idea is that foods from different food groups, when eaten together, don't digest properly and cause toxicity in the stomach, resulting in weight gain and lethargy. If foods are combined in meals in the planned way – for instance not mixing proteins with starches – they digest completely. You feel fitter, brighter and will lose weight – if you need to.

Pros
It is possible to have a perfectly balanced daily diet when using this diet, even though each meal is not correctly balanced. You are unlikely to be hungry as snacks are allowed and there is no calorie counting. It is easy to follow (but see below).

Cons
It takes quite a while to understand the regime and get used to it. It cuts out lots of favourites like jacket potatoes with cheese, Ploughman's lunches, fish and chips and curry with rice!

Effectiveness
There is no scientific evidence to show it works, but many people find they do lose weight – if they follow the rules rigidly. It is designed as a long-term eating plan, not a quick reducing diet. However, it doesn't fit in with normal, social eating, so most people can't stick to it.

High-protein, low-carbohydrate diets

Protein is harder to digest than carbohydrate so if you eat more of it, you burn up more calories processing it and therefore lose weight. In addition, eating large quantities of protein and little carbohydrate will reduce your appetite and will make you lose weight. (This is because the more bulk – carbohydrate – you eat, the more you want and the more you eat.)

Pros

You are unlikely to feel hungry. Portion sizes are unlimited and you don't have to count calories or fat units.

Cons

These diets are seriously low in complex carbohydrates and lack essential vitamins and minerals. Also, eating too much protein produces toxic substances in the body, which can be harmful.

Effectiveness

You are likely to lose weight quickly at first but the regime is not healthy and should not be followed for more than two weeks or you may become ill. When you start eating normally, the weight will return.

Low-fat diets

Fat equals fat – so says the thinking behind this one – so all added fats are removed or drastically reduced, thus causing weight loss.

Pros

It encourages you to eat less saturated fat in your diet – a good idea for most of us. Fruit and vegetables are also encouraged.

Cons

To be healthy, your body must have some essential fats (omega-3 and omega-6 fatty acids) and many low-fat diets ignore this.

Effectiveness

Without the essential fatty acids, the body can't function properly so any weight loss will, by necessity, be short-term and will be reversed when you return to normal eating – as you will have to do sooner or later. A diet that reduces saturated fat is good for everyone but a very low-fat or no-fat diet is definitely not.

Replacement meal diets

One or more meals a day are replaced by special products. These may be either bought shakes or medically supervised plans, such as the Cambridge diet. For over-the-counter diets, you normally have two shakes a day and one low-calorie, low-fat meal. On the medically supervised diets, you eat only the product and no ordinary food for a specified time.

Pros
These diets are easy to follow. The replacement meals are usually fortified with vitamins and minerals so you shouldn't suffer any deficiencies.

Cons
The daily calorie count is very low. It's boring and anti-social and the craving to eat a substantial meal can be overwhelming.

Effectiveness
As soon as you stop, you'll put on weight again. You won't have learned any good eating habits for the future.

Slimming clubs

You sign on as a member of a class and are given special diet sheets to follow. You have to be weighed in public on a regular basis and will be applauded (or not) according to your weight loss. Foods on the diet sheets are categorised into those you can eat in abundance, those that are healthy extras and those that are 'sinful'. You are allowed to earn 'sinful' foods according to how good you've been, in terms of calorie intake.

Pros

There are lots of incentives to succeed. You have actually paid to be a member of a class. The staff and other members provide support. You are unlikely to feel hungry and can have some treats (if you're good most of the time!) Meal plans are nutritionally sound.

Cons

On a psychological level, the idea of some foods being 'sinful' foods is very bad for people who are already hung up about what they are eating. Weight loss will be gradual, not dramatic, which can be frustrating and cause people to give up.

Effectiveness

It's not a 'quick fix'. Weight loss will happen over a period of time if you stick to the regime – and some people do manage it. But most people's will-power ebbs, and then it's back to square one – or beyond.

Slimming pills

There are four types:

Starch blockers prevent the digestion of carbohydrate and so stop you gaining weight.

Fat attackers reduce fat digestion. Fats in the food stick to the chemical in the body, binding with it, and are then passed out of the body. Because you are not absorbing any fat, you'll lose weight.

Appetite suppressants fool your brain into thinking that your stomach is full, so you eat less and lose weight.

Diuretics make your body get rid of fluids. They stimulate the kidneys to work overtime, excreting urine. Fluid equals weight, so your weight drops off.

Pros

You can just carry on eating as normal, believing the pills will do the work for you.

Cons

Starch blockers have unpleasant side effects, such as bacterial and yeast infections of the gut and serious flatulence.

Fat attackers are a bad idea: it is essential that your body absorbs some fats (see page 19, Low-fat Diets). A fat deficiency can mean tiredness, mood swings and dry hair, nails and skin.

Appetite suppressants are actually stimulants. These and diuretics can cause numerous side effects including headaches, dehydration, anxiety and lack of co-ordination. They will also ruin your body's natural metabolism.

Effectiveness
Slimming pills are not the answer. You may have an initial weight loss but this may, in turn, lead to rapid weight gain, serious eating disorders and even liver, kidney or heart failure.

Chapter 2
Healthy Eating for Life

Ultimately, your purpose should be to establish a new eating regime, so that you can not only lose weight but also permanently maintain that weight loss while still enjoying yourself.

Our food is made up of many different items, but I have divided it into five main groups. In order to feel good, look good and remain fit and healthy, it is important that you eat foods from all five of these food groups every day in suitable quantities. As we have already seen, many diets are deficient in one or more elements – but not this one. In Chapter 6, Your 28-day Diet Plan, on pages 65–94, I have given you a reducing diet, with every meal carefully planned and laid out, to ensure that you will be getting the right balance without having to think about it. By the time you move on to Chapter 8, Maintaining the New You, healthy eating will be second nature and easy to achieve.

The five food groups you need to bear in mind are described in detail on the following pages.

Cereals, grains and potatoes

These are starchy foods (carbohydrates) that provide fuel to give you the energy to do everything from sleeping and thinking to running a marathon. They will also fill you up and keep you warm. Half of what you eat every day should come from this group. That is potatoes, yams, sweet potatoes, pasta, rice, oats and other grains, polenta, couscous, bulghar, every type of bread and breakfast cereals.

You are probably putting your hands up in horror and saying 'But eating all that will make me fat!' Trust me, it won't – it's the oodles of butter, other fats and sugary products you pile on to them that will do the damage. The starches on my list are essential to health.

Fruit and vegetables

The more fruit and vegetables you eat, the better your health and well-being. They provide essential vitamins, minerals and fibre and help prevent heart disease and cancer. They are also low in calories so are ideal snack foods.

This group includes every type of fruit and vegetable you can imagine – they can be fresh, frozen, dried, canned in natural juice or water (not oil or syrup) and pure fruit and vegetable juices (but not fruit drinks, which contain masses of sugar and other additives). You should aim to consume at least five portions a day. (A portion is a piece of fruit, a glass of pure juice or an average serving of vegetables.)

Proteins

Proteins are vital for the growth and repair of all body tissue. You'll find them in red meat, such as lamb, pork, beef and venison, in poultry, fish and eggs, and in vegetable sources like dried peas, beans and lentils, nuts, tofu and Quorn. You don't need very much protein in your daily diet – about 10–15 per cent of your total food intake is enough – but it is important to eat a variety of foods within the group, so I would suggest you have two or three small portions of different proteins each day.

Dairy products

Milk, cheese and yoghurt all contain calcium, which is necessary for healthy teeth and bones. If you don't get enough, you may be vulnerable to osteoporosis (brittle bones) in later life as well as having rotten teeth. If you don't want to eat dairy products or can't tolerate them, you can get enough calcium from enriched soya milk, dried figs and apricots and green leafy vegetables like spinach and spring (collard) greens. As a guide, each day you will need the equivalent of 600 ml/1 pt/2½ cups skimmed milk, or a generous chunk (about 25 g/1 oz) of reduced-fat Cheddar cheese, or two small pots of yoghurt.

Fats and sugars

Essential fats (omega-3 and omega-6 fatty acids) are vital for the function of our nervous system, and to keep your nails, hair and skin healthy. These are found naturally in foods in the other groups and your body doesn't need any extra in your diet, so keep added fats to a minimum – they are loaded with calories. Have just a scraping of reduced-fat olive or sunflower spread on bread, use the minimum of sunflower or olive oil in cooking and avoid all saturated animal fats: cut off fat on meat, remove the skin from chicken and so on.

Natural sugars are a good source of energy and are found in fruit, vegetables and grains. You don't need added sugar; it's loaded with calories and will make you fat with no added benefits. Keep it to a minimum, having sweet, sugary foods as treats rather than filling up on them.

Fluids

In addition to solid food, it is vital that your body gets enough water as it is the basis of every bodily function. You need at least 2 litres/3½ pts/8½ cups of fluid a day. This doesn't have to be pure water; it's in everything you drink, from milk to pure juice, tea to beer.

Remember, though, sugary drinks and alcohol are high in calories. Choose low-calorie diet alternatives. If you want alcohol, it should be limited to two to three units a day for women, three to four for men (I shall explain later how to incorporate them in the plan). Drinks that contain caffeine, like tea and coffee, act as a stimulant only if drunk in moderation. If you have too much you may stop your body from absorbing essential vitamins and minerals and you will begin to feel sluggish.

Finding your perfect weight

You know in your heart when you are overweight. Your clothes feel tight and don't hang properly, or you have to buy a larger size than you did previously. When you stand in front of the mirror without clothes, you see rolls of flab where, maybe, you were once firm – or at least only gently curving. Your stomach appears swollen even if you try hard to draw it in, you have more than one chin and your face appears puffy. Whether you have only a few pounds to lose or a lot more to deal with, it's time to take action.

Check Your Weight

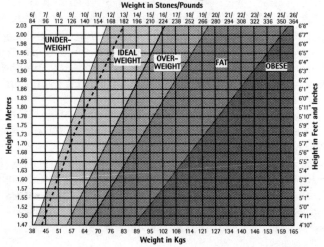

The first thing to do is establish exactly how much you need to lose. The chart on page 28, based on UK government statistics, shows you how much you should weigh according to your height. Your weight depends on your bone structure, so you may be at the lower end of the scale or higher up. The important thing is to be within the limits of your ideal weight.

Having discovered these limits, weigh yourself first thing in the morning, preferably without clothes. (If you weigh yourself with any clothes on, make sure you wear similar attire each time you check your weight). Compare your actual weight with your ideal weight on the chart, then work out how much weight you need to lose. Once you've made that calculation and started your diet, you should weigh yourself in the same way, using the same scales, **once a week only**. There is usually a quick burst of weight loss in the first few days, and then it will level off. But at the end of a month you will have a significant and sustainable weight loss in a painless way.

Sneaky Ways to Make Weight Loss Easier

Dieting is never easy but there are lots of ways to make it more bearable.

- Use a smaller plate for meals.
- Drink lots of water. A glass of naturally sparkling mineral water will help fill you up in between, before and with your meals (zip it up with a slice of lemon or lime if you like).

- Cut foods into smaller pieces or thinner slices. Have the same number of pieces/slices as normal – you'll think you've had the same but you'll actually have had less.
- Chew slowly and eat small forkfuls. Your meal will last longer.
- Try to eat meals before you're ravenously hungry – especially if you are going to a restaurant!
- Never go shopping on an empty stomach – it's too tempting.
- In a restaurant, choose a starter and main course that are low in calories. They will fill you up without doing too much damage to your diet and you will be more inclined to avoid the calorie-packed desserts.
- Eat as many vegetables or salad stuffs as you like – but not laced with oil or melted butter.
- If you feel really peckish between meals, eat some raw carrots or any salad vegetables, a bunch of grapes or an apple to keep you going and take the edge off your appetite.
- A hot drink made with meat or yeast extract (Bovril or Marmite) – a teaspoonful to a mug of boiling water – is another good way to take the edge off your appetite or fill up between meals.
- Avoid adding sugar to your food, including cereals and drinks. Use artificial sweetener if you have to and sweeten sour fruits like rhubarb with a little honey. You'll need less than if you used sugar but don't be tempted to add more than is absolutely necessary.
- Choose low-calorie brands of soft drinks, dressings, etc.

- Choose canned fruits in natural juice, not syrup, and canned fish in brine, not oil, where available.
- Drink unsweetened pure fruit juices (but beware the cartons of 'fruit juice drinks' – they contain sugar and other additives).
- Check labels of so-called 'reduced-fat' products. Some have more calories than regular brands because they often contain more sugar.
- Keep a packet of sugar-free chewing gum handy and chew between meals.
- If you feel like grabbing a handful of nuts, clean your teeth instead – it really works!
- Always take the trouble to make your meal look appetising. A sprinkling of parsley or some vegetables attractively arranged will help you enjoy what you're eating.
- Avoid cooking in fat – grill (broil) instead wherever possible. Use only the minimum of oil or low-fat spread suitable for cooking, and only where absolutely necessary. When browning meat for a made-up dish, dry-fry and then spoon off any fat (but keep the juices). Cut any excess fat off meat before and after cooking and remove skin from poultry. For lots more ways of cutting down your fat intake, see page 48.
- **Don't cheat!** You know if you are piling food on your plate when you should be being less-than-generous. Just remember, the smaller the portion, the more you'll lose.

You will find lots more tips on pages 46–53.

Chapter 3
Wise Ways to Weight Reduction

We all know that by eating a healthy diet and taking regular exercise (not necessarily frenetic, but at least 30 minutes a day of physical activity, such as walking, gardening or swimming), we can achieve a sensible body weight. We also know that it may help prevent heart disease and diet-related illnesses like diabetes. But if you are overweight, finding the right diet is not always easy, especially when there are so many cranky ones around. Take another look at Chapter 2 to see a breakdown of some of the different ones available and why they don't work in the long term – you'll see what I mean.

Being overweight or obese can be depressing – especially when we are surrounded by svelte role models. But, more importantly, it is seriously damaging to your health. There is no secret as to how the problem arises: it is quite simply because you put more fuel (calories) into your body than you burn up. The excess calories are stored as fat, on the hips and thighs in women and around the stomach in men. Obviously, the more excess fat you have, the wider it spreads, so your chest, legs, arms and shoulders will also continue to enlarge as you store more and more fat.

So, for the sake of your health and your future, you need to take action – and it needs to be action that works!

It is pointless putting yourself on a starvation diet, depriving yourself of everything you enjoy – like chocolate, cakes or the odd glass of wine. Your will-power will dwindle very quickly, and even though you will initially lose weight, you won't maintain that loss. And if the diet is extremely low in calories, you will become ill and look dreadful. Your body has to have enough 'fuel' and nutrients to stay healthy.

Ideally, you should aim to lose up to 1 kg/1–2 lb a week. This will mean reducing your intake to 1,000–1,200 calories a day if you are a woman, 1,300–1,500 if you are a man. However, be warned, our bodies being what they are, your weight loss will 'plateau' after a few weeks (whether you are snacking or not). When this happens, don't despair: keep going. Your body will readjust and, providing you keep a good balance of nutrients (eating what you should eat according to the diet plan including the allowed snacks, and **not cheating**), you will start to lose again. Then, once you've reached your goal, you can maintain your new shape effortlessly, following some very simple guidelines.

More than just cutting down on calories

As I've already said, if you're going to get your body down to the size you want, you can't rely solely on what you consume. The diet will make you lose weight but you need to think about how you spend the rest of your time when you're not eating and drinking to maintain long-term success and a new slender you.

Starting on page 40 there is a questionnaire that will tell you about your eating habits. This is followed by specific advice on how to achieve a healthier lifestyle. But you have to realise that exercise is vital in burning off calories and toning the muscles. Don't panic, I'm not proposing you have a regimented exercise programme where you have to spend ages every day puffing, panting and contorting – you probably wouldn't keep it up after the first day or two! Instead, think about putting the things you do daily to good use, to tone your body, get your heart pumping and create a new, healthier you. Every physical movement you make, from blinking your eyes to going on a long run, burns up calories. Obviously, the more strenuous the activity, the more you use up. And, even when you aren't doing anything that takes any effort – like watching television – you can trim your tummy, tone up your leg muscles and use up a few more calories than you might imagine. Just spend a few minutes each day doing the non-intrusive exercises on pages 35–37. Do them at least once a day – more if you like! In addition, try to make regular, more strenuous exercise part of your daily life.

Non-intrusive exercising

There is no need to buy expensive equipment, go to the gym or join a special class to do exercises. You can tone your body any time, whatever you're doing – lying in the bath, watching TV, preparing the vegetables for dinner or sitting in a traffic jam.

Facial toning

Head side tilts: Keeping your shoulders down, tip your head gently to the right so your ear is close to your shoulder, then straighten. Do the same to the left. Keep your shoulders still. Repeat 8 times.

Chin tilts: Keeping your shoulders down, bend your head so your chin rests on your chest and you feel the stretch in the back of your neck. Slowly lift your head up to your normal position, then tilt back so you feel the stretch under your chin. Slowly return to normal. Repeat 8 times.

Head circle: Start with your chin on your chest, then gently rotate your head so you look over your right shoulder, then slowly lift your head up so you are looking upwards, then back to chin on chest. Repeat, looking over your left shoulder. Repeat 4 times each way.

The surprise: Pucker your mouth, then gradually open it as wide as you can, drawing your lips back and opening and lifting your eyebrows at the same time. You should feel the skin stretch all round your face. (Beware of doing this in public, as you may get some strange looks!) Repeat 8 times.

Limbering up

The shrug: Keep your head still. With your arms by your sides or folded in your lap, raise your shoulders slowly up under your ears, then release slowly. Repeat 8 times.

Shoulder circles: Keeping your head still, raise your shoulders up under your ears, then pull the shoulder blades back and down, then tilt them forward, then up under your ears and back down in a backward circular movement. Repeat 8 times.

Tummy tone: Sit upright with your shoulders down, hands loosely in your lap, or stand in a relaxed position if you prefer. Breathe in deeply, pulling in your tummy muscles towards your backbone. Hold for the count of three, then breathe out and relax. Repeat 8 times.

The secret clench: Again, do this sitting or standing. Clench your pelvic floor muscles (as if you are stopping yourself urinating). Hold for the count of three and release. Repeat 8 times.

The bottom raiser: Clench your buttocks tightly together and draw in your pelvic floor muscles at the same time. Hold for the count of three and release. If you're sitting down, you should feel yourself rise up and down as you clench and release. Repeat 8 times.

Hands and feet stretch: Screw your fists up, then slowly stretch out your fingers as far as they will go, so you feel the skin stretch across your palms. Do the same thing with your feet, curling and then stretching your toes. Repeat 8 times.

Wrist turns: Hold your hands in front of you, fingers together, palms down. Gently rotate your wrists by circling your hands, still keeping the palms downwards. Do this 4 times one way, then 4 times the other.

Ankle turns: With your legs outstretched, lift one leg just off the floor and gently rotate the ankle in a circle first one way, then back the other way. Repeat with the other ankle. Repeat 8 times.

Exercise as part of your life

If you're keen on going to the gym or doing aerobics, you've got this cracked. But if not, there are plenty of ways you can take regular exercise without it being a major undertaking.

- Walk instead of using the car or public transport whenever possible. Always walk at a brisk pace instead of wandering along.
- If you take the bus, get off a stop before your usual one and walk the last part of the journey.
- Ride a bike if you have one.
- Get into the habit of using the stairs instead of lifts or escalators.
- Take up a recreational sport like tennis or swimming or join a dance class – or just go clubbing/dancing regularly.
- If you have a garden, enjoy working in it. If you live in a flat, get an allotment (or offer to help in a friend's garden). Half an hour's weeding the garden will burn up over 100 calories!

Bending and stretching exercises will, of course, help to tone your muscles but you must do them properly or you can cause yourself damage. Seek advice before you start any kind of exercise programme. If you are going to exercise at home, make it a regular part of your daily routine, perhaps before you have your shower or bath in the morning or evening, so it becomes as natural as brushing your teeth. If you don't, the novelty will wear off after a few days and you won't persevere.

How many calories do you burn?

Here's a list of various daily activities to give you an idea of how much energy you burn. The more strenuous the activity, the more energy you need, and so the more calories you burn. For instance, if you spend 15 minutes driving to the shops, you'll burn only around 30 calories. But dig the garden for the same amount of time and you'll use up around 120 calories.

Activity	Calories/15 minutes
Aerobics	105
Ballroom dancing	90
Climbing stairs	165
Cycling, fast or uphill	165
Cycling, leisurely speed	60
Disco dancing	105
Driving a car	30
Gardening, digging	120

Activity	Calories/15 minutes
Gardening, hoeing	60
Golf	60
Gym work-out	105
Hill-walking	120
Horse-riding, hacking	30
Horse-riding, trotting and cantering	90
House work	60
Jogging	90
Manual work, heavy	120
Manual work, light	60
Running, fast	105
Shopping	60
Sleeping	15
Squash	135
Swimming, racing speed	150
Swimming, relaxed speed	105
Tennis	140
Typing	30
Walking, relaxed speed	60
Walking, briskly	105
Watching TV	15

Chapter 4
Lifestyle Quiz

I t is vital that the diet plan you use suits you. I have designed this quiz for you to find out how healthy your lifestyle is, where your weaknesses lie and, most important, how to overcome them.

Answer all the questions in this section as honestly as you can, selecting the answers closest to your own lifestyle.

1   **What sort of breakfast do you have?**
   (a) I grab a coffee and sometimes a slice of toast on my way out of the door.
   (b) I have a hearty meal, sometimes cooked.
   (c) I never eat breakfast.
   (d) I have a light meal, like juice and cereal and/or toast.

2   **If you feel peckish during the morning or afternoon, what do you have?**
   (a) A biscuit (cookie), a packet of crisps (potato chips) or a chocolate bar.
   (b) A substantial snack, like a cheese roll.
   (c) I never eat snacks between meals.
   (d) A piece of fruit.

3 **At lunchtime what sort of food do you have?**
   (a) A cooked meal, either at home or in a restaurant, canteen or pub.
   (b) A filling snack, like a pork pie, a packet of crisps and a chocolate biscuit.
   (c) I skip lunch.
   (d) A light meal, like a sandwich or a salad and fruit.

4 **What do you normally eat for your main meal?**
   (a) A supermarket cook/chill meal.
   (b) A take-away.
   (c) A restaurant meal.
   (d) A home-cooked meal.

5 **How much alcohol do you drink a day?**
   (A unit of alcohol is 300 ml/½ pt of ordinary-strength beer, a glass of wine or a single measure of spirits)
   (a) More than 3 units.
   (b) 2–3 units.
   (c) I don't drink.
   (d) 1–2 units.

6 **How often do you eat chocolate?**
   (a) At least once a day.
   (b) Several times a week.
   (c) I don't eat chocolate.
   (d) Occasionally.

7 **How many portions of fruit and vegetables do you eat in a day?**
(A portion is a piece of fruit; a glass of pure fruit or vegetable juice or an average serving of a vegetable, salad or canned or small soft fruit, such as strawberries.)
(a) 3–4 portions.
(b) 1–2 portions.
(c) I hardly eat any at all.
(d) 5 or more portions.

8 **What means of transport do you usually use?**
(a) I cycle.
(b) I travel by car.
(c) I take public transport.
(d) I walk most places.

9 **When you're feeling depressed or unhappy what do you do?**
(a) I drink alcohol or eat chocolates.
(b) I eat a cream cake (or similar).
(c) I go off my food.
(d) None of these.

10 **What is your ideal way of spending an evening with friends?**
(a) A few drinks down the pub.
(b) A take-away and a video.
(c) A restaurant meal.
(d) A dinner party at home.

11 What sort of exercise do you do regularly?
(At least once a week)
(a) I work out at a gym/go to an aerobics or keep-fit class.
(b) I do little or no exercise.
(c) I rush around a lot every day as part of my job/lifestyle.
(d) I play active sport (e.g. tennis, squash, swimming, netball, hockey, football).

12 What is your favourite hobby?
(a) Dancing/clubbing.
(b) Gardening/DIY etc.
(c) The arts, e.g. books, music, theatre, films, TV.
(d) Playing sports.

13 Which of these best describes the way you sleep?
(a) I have no trouble going to sleep but wake after a couple of hours.
(b) I take ages to get to sleep.
(c) I am a very light sleeper.
(d) I sleep soundly.

14 Which of these best describes your temperament?
(a) Sometimes stressed.
(b) Laid-back.
(c) Shy.
(d) Confident.

15 What do you think of your naked body … honestly?
(a) Hips, thighs and/or stomach are too big.
(b) Very overweight – everywhere.
(c) Flabby.
(d) Rounded where I don't want to be.

15 Which of these best describes your personality?
(a) Friendly, extroverted.
(b) Easy-going.
(c) Quiet, introverted.
(d) Practical, happy.

16 If you were going to a party and driving, what would you drink?
(a) I can drink loads of alcohol without it affecting me, so I have what I feel like.
(b) Three alcoholic drinks because that's how much you're allowed before being over the limit.
(c) Just one alcoholic drink, then soft drinks.
(d) Soft drinks – I never drink and drive/I don't drink.

17 How would you describe your eating habits?
(a) I eat when I'm hungry, not at specific times.
(b) I eat too much.
(c) I hardly eat a thing but still put on weight.
(d) I eat three square meals a day.

18 **What would you choose from a restaurant dessert trolley?**
   (a) Chocolate fudge cake.
   (b) Cheese and biscuits.
   (c) Ice cream.
   (d) Fresh fruit salad.

19 **When you go on a reducing diet, what is your worst problem?**
   (a) Having to deprive myself of favourite treats, like chocolate or booze – I just crave for them even more.
   (b) Feeling hungry.
   (c) Trying to fit the diet into my lifestyle.
   (d) I miss eating 'proper' food.

20 **What part does food play in your life?**
   (a) I hate cooking but enjoy eating.
   (b) I live to eat – food and more food please!
   (c) I eat to live – it is a necessary but uninteresting part of my existence.
   (d) I love cooking and good food.

Now go through your replies and add up how many (a)s, (b)s, (c)s and (d)s you scored.

How did you rate?

Obviously none of us is so stereotyped that we fall exactly into any one category. This is just a fun guide to give you an idea of the way you might think about food, your body and your lifestyle. It may tell you a few home truths or you may know them already. Either way, it'll give you some useful dieting tips and the incentive to go on and follow the perfect diet for you!

Mostly (a)s

You enjoy life to the full. You indulge yourself and can't resist temptation. You are likely to have little or no will-power and need this diet because it will allow you to still have your booze, chocolate and other little treats to keep you going. If you feel you are sometimes a bit excessive, this diet will help you keep things in moderation (but not in a boring way), leading to a healthier, happier you.

Ways to control your indulgences:

Alcohol: If you can't cut down on the number of drinks you have a day, have smaller glasses. That way the quantity of alcohol and the calories will be reduced (to stick to the diet plan you'll have to allow yourself no more than the recommended intake). If you drink beer, choose an ordinary-strength one – there are 120 calories more in a 300 ml/½ pt glass of high-strength variety! Always choose low-calorie mixers. Have single, not double, measures. Choose dry instead of sweet drinks. Sip them and put the glass down between sips.

Chocolate: Don't buy big blocks, jumbo bags or boxes of chocolates. The temptation to go on eating is too great. Buy only what you are allowed to eat in a week (see Snack Attack on page 56) so you aren't tempted to eat any more. Tell the rest of the family or other people in your household what you're doing so they can help guard against cheating!

Sweets and biscuits (candy and cookies): Again, don't buy big packets of sweets, or, ideally, don't buy them at all! Have packets of sugar-free gum to chew when you have a craving (or, if you really can't do without them, choose sugar-free sweets (a sugar-free lollipop can be sucked for quite a long time to satisfy that craving). Be careful though, the sorbitol in sugar-free sweets can lead to an upset tummy if you eat too much!

If you can't resist biscuits, try to buy plain varieties rather than chocolate-coated or cream-filled. You're allowed two plain ones but only one cream-filled as a snack but in the long term, it's best to check the calorie count on each packet and go for the lowest you can find – a Rich Tea, for instance, is only 39 calories whereas a Bourbon Cream is 63 calories! Don't be fooled by those labels with 'low-fat' claims. They may well be lower in fat but are likely to be higher in sugar to compensate so may be no better calorie-wise.

Mostly (b)s

You are likely to be quite overweight. You have a high-fat/high-calorie diet so you need to start cutting down **now**. Diets probably don't usually work for you because you feel hungry so you give up or you cheat, kidding yourself you are eating the quantities recommended when you know you are piling up your plate or slapping butter on your bread with a trowel. My diet plan will be ideal for you. It will help you cut down on fat and calories effortlessly while still keeping you feeling full and satisfied.

To help you cut down on fat:

- Choose the lowest-fat diet dairy products (yoghurts, cheeses, cream, etc.) you can find (read the labels).
- Use a low-fat spread instead of butter or conventional margarine.
- Have only a scraping of low-fat spread on bread and don't add it to vegetables.
- Beware of hot toast and newly baked bread – they just cry out for thick dollops of butter and even if you use low-fat spread, it will melt in, inviting you to add more.
- Keep some of your low-fat spread at room temperature (but don't keep all of it out of the fridge all the time as it doesn't keep as well as full-fat varieties). It will spread much more easily, so you will use far less, saving up to half the calories. For example, a slice of bread and low-fat spread straight from the fridge is 117 calories, but spread thinly with warmer spread it will be only 98 calories!

- Use a strong-flavoured cheese in cooking – you won't need so much to give it a good flavour.
- Drink skimmed milk rather than semi-skimmed or whole milk.
- Choose lean meats and trim off excess fat, preferably before cooking if possible.
- Remove all fat or skin from meat and poultry before eating.

Mostly (c)s

You probably think you've only got to look at food and you put on weight. The chances are that in reality you don't eat balanced meals, nibble a lot (without even realising it) and don't really enjoy what you eat. This diet will help you eat properly without making you eat big meals if you don't want to (see the tips on page 50 for eating little and often instead of full meals, if you prefer) and will help you take pleasure in your food. You'll feel better about yourself in every way. Also, in the past you may have found diets hard because you have other people to feed and you don't want to have different food from them. My diet is ideal because all the food is 'normal' and suitable for everyone.

First you need to discover ways to achieve a healthy balance without eating big meals. Start by noting for a day exactly what you do eat – you may be surprised. I don't mean just your meals, I mean **everything** that passes your lips, from a cup of coffee with full-cream milk to a cold potato left in the fridge. It will probably be obvious that, despite not eating big meals, you are consuming far more than you imagined.

To help you cut down:
- Put snacks from the 1-point list (see page 62) into containers and keep them handy so you can nibble those instead of the leftovers in the fridge.
- Change to the lower-calorie options for things like full-cream milk and, generally, start to think before you pop things into your mouth!
- Drink pure fruit juice or vegetable juice instead of squash or carbonated drinks.
- Get your five portions of fruit and vegetables by nibbling them between meals.
- Cut up pieces of fruit or vegetables (like carrots, cucumber, radishes or celery) and keep them in the fridge or in a plastic box at work to nibble when you're peckish. Alternatively eat a handful of raisins or other dried fruits (see my 1-point Snacks on page 62).
- Avoid nibbling other people's leftovers (particularly when the children leave half of their tea).

To help you balance your diet:
- If you hate fruit and vegetables, try these tips to get your quota each day. Make a pot of soup by simmering any selection of vegetables in some chicken or vegetable stock with a pinch of dried mixed herbs and a little seasoning until soft. Purée the soup in a blender or food processor until smooth, then cool and store it in the fridge. Heat up at least one mugful a day. For a change, try making a cold soup –

again, you should have at least one mugful per day. Cook some carrots and purée them with canned tomatoes, red or green (bell) peppers, some cucumber and a tiny bit of onion. Flavour with a pinch of dried herbs, a squeeze of lemon and some salt and pepper. Keep in the fridge.

- If you can't face a big meal, have a sandwich with just a scraping of low-fat spread, filled with salad and a small amount of one of the following: lean meat, fish (like tuna in brine, canned salmon, mashed sardines, crab or prawns), reduced-fat cheese, egg or mashed, canned pulses. This will give you a perfectly balanced meal instead any of the main courses in the diet.
- Try to sit down when you eat your food.
- Make your meal look attractive – it's surprising what a sprig of parsley or a colourful choice of vegetables, nicely arranged, can do for the taste buds.
- Eat with other people, if possible. It makes the meal a social event rather than a chore.
- Rearrange what you eat and when. If the complete meal suggested in my diet plan seems too much, have, for instance, the main course at your mealtime and the pudding suggestion a couple of hours later.
- Try taking more regular exercise – as well as keeping you fit, it will boost your appetite for proper meals.

Mostly (d)s

You have a relatively healthy lifestyle so you probably wonder why you are overweight. It's simply that you are consuming more calories than you are burning in a day. My diet is ideal for you. It will help you regulate your food intake while still maintaining a healthy balance. You'll be trim and svelte in no time!

Ways to reduce your daily quantity of food:

- Have a glass of sparkling water before you eat.
- Use a smaller plate.
- Don't have second helpings.
- Have your usual number of slices of meats, cheese, bread, etc., but choose thin slices.
- Avoid too many oily dressings and go for low-calorie options of mayonnaise, etc.
- Choose reduced-sugar preserves.
- Don't add butter or other fat to vegetables at the table. Buy a low-fat spread and use it very sparingly on bread.
- Increase the amount of exercise you do.

Fairly evenly split between two options – e.g. similar total of (a)s and (d)s

Read both the results. Like being on the cusp of a star sign, you may find you are a bit of both categories, so both sets of help points may be of use!

A complete mixture of (a)s, (b)s, (c)s and (d)s

The chances are you are quite an erratic sort of person and this is reflected in your weight. Sometimes you feel okay about it, sometimes you feel fat and your actual weight probably fluctuates as well, perhaps quite drastically.

It's time for action. No more eating loads of chocolate biscuits (cookies) one day because you feel down, then going on a fast for a few days to compensate. You gain weight because your body is not fed properly so it doesn't function to its optimum and your metabolism is unstable. You need to take control and start to eat more healthily and sensibly.

Tackling the issues:

- Do not skip any meals. If you haven't got time or don't feel like any meal, make a Smoothie for breakfast (see Breakfast Options, page 63) and the soups I suggested on page 50 for lunch or supper. Alternatively, drink a can of vegetable juice, or a large glass of skimmed milk. It's not ideal, but it's better than missing meals completely. This is so important I can't stress it enough.

- On days when you're down and tempted to eat a whole packet of chocolate biscuits, stop and think. Drink a glass of sparkling water, wait five minutes, have one biscuit, as allowed in your diet and concentrate on something active and practical like cleaning out a cupboard, doing the filing, or taking the dog for a walk. Whatever you do, don't sit down with a cup of coffee and a book – the biscuit tin will be out again in a flash!

- Once you're into the diet and eating sensibly every day, you can make those treats psychologically important. Earmark them for parts of the day when you know you'll need them. For example, it may be that you usually have a drink when you come in from work. Okay, save enough points (by not eating all those biscuits!) to really look forward to that drink. But don't just have it automatically while you prepare supper – sit down and enjoy it.
- Read the points in all the other answers, as many of them will also apply to you!

This diet can work wonders. Follow it faithfully and within the month your body's metabolism will be working superbly and you'll feel so much better in yourself.

Chapter 5
Using the Diet Plan

This book contains a complete, 28-day diet plan. You'll have three meals a day, which you can prepare yourself from the recipes at the back of the book or you can use ready-made meals if you prefer. My unique Snack Attack feature includes some favourite treats in your diet. Please note: you must eat all the fruit and vegetables – if you don't, the diet simply won't work. So if you hate 'eating up your greens', see my suggestions on page 50 of the Lifestyle Quiz for alternative ways of getting them inside you. Also, breakfast is a must. If you can't face eating it, see my suggestions on page 63.

Men on the diet 🕴

I have made special allowances for men on my diet plan. This is not sexist, it's just a fact of life: men need more calories a day than women so they can have extra carbohydrates during the diet. This is not just because men tend to be taller, it is because they have a higher metabolic rate and store fat in a different way. The men's allowances are clearly marked 🕴 throughout the plan. You can either have more of the listed item, in which case the quantity is indicated in brackets – (🕴 4) – or sometimes you can have a little something extra!

Snack attack

This is what makes my diet plan really different and the best ever! This diet enables you to have the treats that make life worthwhile, together with your balanced, nutritious calorie-controlled diet. You are allowed up to 6 points-worth of extras a day. But remember, the fewer you eat, the quicker you'll lose weight, so you don't **have** to have the treats at all!

You will see that the snacks are listed in categories. The most calorific are in the 6-point list. The fairly high-calorie counts are in the 4-point list, the reasonable ones are in the 2-point list and the low-calorie ones, which are to be positively encouraged, are in the 1-point list.

Every day you must eat all your meals. Then you can have up to 6 points-worth of snacks. Do not have snacks instead of any part of the meal – especially the fruit or vegetables, they are intended to be eaten **as well as** your meals. If you can't stand fruit and vegetables, follow the guidelines on page 50 of the Lifestyle Quiz. The quick-lose way is to have no extras at all, of course, and the healthy option is to take all your snacks from the 1-point section.

So, for instance you can have just one 6-point snack and nothing else. This means that if you elect to have a chocolate éclair, you can't have wine as well. But if you decide to have a Flake chocolate bar (4 points), you could also have a glass of wine (2 points). Alternatively, you can 'save up' snacks. So, for instance, if you are having a special meal on a Saturday night and know you want nibbles with drinks, more wine **and** a high-calorie dessert, make sure you have enough points left from the day before to allow for it.

Do not cheat. Don't have larger snacks than allowed (such as a family bar of chocolate instead of an individual standard bar, or 'top-ups' of wine). Also, if you have a double gin and tonic or other spirit, it counts as double (i.e. 4 points, not 2). Just remember, if you kid yourself, you won't succeed.

Chocolate bars are all standard size, i.e. one up from fun size, and packets of sweets (candies) are all small, i.e. about 50 g/2 oz. Cakes, ice creams and desserts are all individual size, and slices are average – be sensible! Crisps (potato chips), nuts and savoury snacks are small packets, i.e. 25 g/1 oz.

6-point snacks
Sweets (candy) and chocolate

Boost bar	Maltesers
Bounty bar	Mars Bar
Chocolate bar	M & Ms
Chocolate raisins	Minstrels
Chocolate peanuts	Peanut brittle
Chocolate Turkish Delight bar	Toffee Crisp
Creme egg	Toffee apple
Drifter bar	Topic bar
Kit Kat Chunky	Walnut whip

Biscuits (cookies) and cakes

American (e.g blueberry) muffin
Bakewell tart
Bath bun
Belgian bun
Cheesecake
Chocolate éclair
Cream bun
Doughnut (any flavour)
Eccles cake
Fruit or mince pie
Fruit flan
Sponge cake

Ice creams and desserts

'99'
Bounty ice cream
Choc ice
Chocolate dessert with cream
Chocolate roulade
Cornetto
Magnum
Mars ice cream
Tiramisu
Topic ice cream
Twix ice cream
Viennetta or ice cream gateau

Savoury snacks

Corn puffs
Corn/ tortilla chips e.g. Doritos
Microwave chips (fries)

Drinks

Small glass of high-strength beer/lager
Mug of drinking chocolate or malted drink, made with semi-skimmed milk
Standard-size extra-thick milkshake
Wineglass of Gaelic (or other liqueur) coffee

4-point snacks

Sweets (candies) and chocolate
Cereal bar (crunchy or chewy)
Fudge finger bar
Flake bar

Milky Way
Tube of fruit gums/pastilles

Biscuits (cookies) and cakes
Chocolate-coated biscuit,
    e.g. Club, Kit Kat, Rocky,
    Penguin, Twix
Fairy cake

French fancy (fondant)
Jam (conserve) or lemon
    curd tart
Macaroon

Ice cream and desserts
Calippo
Ice cream cone, any flavour
    (single scoop)
Crème caramel

Chocolate dessert without
    cream
Chocolate mousse

Savoury snacks
Cheeselets
Crisps (potato chips), any flavour

Peanuts or other roasted nuts
Twiglets

Drinks
Small glass of cider
Glass of Champagne
Cappuccino
Café latte
Single measure of gin/vodka/rum and orange, blackcurrant or
    lime cordial
Single gin and Martini (sweet or dry)
Glass of Pimms
Mug of drinking (sweetened) chocolate, made with skimmed
    milk
A milk shake (about 250 ml/8 fl oz/1 cup), made with skimmed
    or semi-skimmed milk

2-point snacks
Sweets (candies) and chocolates

6 jelly babies
10 Matchmakers
A stick of candy floss
2 chocolate brazils

2 filled chocolates from a box
2 mint chocolates
4 toffees, wrapped

Biscuits (cookies) and cakes
1 Jaffa cake
2 plain biscuits e.g. Rich Tea
1 cream-filled biscuit
    e.g. Bourbon or Jammy Dodger

2 chocolate chip cookies
1 half-coated chocolate biscuit e.g. chocolate digestive
Chocolate crispie cake

Savoury snacks
1 individual Baby Bel cheese
4 Cheddars, or other cheese thins
6 cheese footballs
3 cheese straws
A small finger (no more than 20 g/¾ oz) of low-fat cheese
4 cheese and pineapple chunks on sticks
A handful of pretzels

Ice creams
Fruit ice lolly, any flavour
Ice cream-filled fruit lolly e.g. Mivvi/Split

Drinks
Single rum and mixer, e.g. Bacardi and coke
Single gin/vodka and tonic
Single whisky and ginger/soda/coke
Single measure of spirit, e.g. brandy or whisky, on its own
Single measure of liqueur
Mug of low-calorie drinking (sweetened) chocolate
Small glass of port
Small glass of sherry
Small glass of vermouth, sweet or dry
Glass of wine, red, white or rosé

1-point snacks
An apple
A small bunch of grapes
A large carrot, cut into sticks
Celery (as much as you like)
A bowl of cherries (25)
A kiwi fruit
A large wedge of melon
Lettuce, other salad greens or shredded white cabbage, dressed
     with lemon juice or balsamic vinegar and black pepper (as
     much as you like)
A nectarine
Olives, black or green (8)
A peach
A pear
A handful of ready-to-eat dried prunes/apricots (5)
A small punnet of strawberries, raspberries, blackberries

Breakfast options

Breakfast is important and you should not miss it, although I realise you might not want to have the ideas I've suggested. If you normally skip breakfast altogether and can't face anything very substantial, try the smoothie below. If you don't want to drink it first thing, put it in a bottle, take it to work and drink it when you arrive.

Breakfast smoothie

1 large banana
15 ml/1 tbsp oat or wheat bran
5 ml/1 tsp clear honey
200 ml/7 fl oz/scant 1 cup skimmed milk

Just put all the ingredients in a blender and whisk them together. You can ring the changes by using a small banana and adding a handful of fresh strawberries or raspberries, a ripe peach or nectarine or a couple of plums – remove the stones (pits) first, of course!

If you only ever eat cereal for breakfast, have a small glass of pure fruit juice and either a bowl of corn flakes, branflakes – plain or with sultanas (golden raisins) or All-bran, or 1 (♀ 2) Weetabix or Shredded Wheat, with skimmed milk.

If you must sweeten cereal, tea or coffee, use an artificial granular sweetener – but, ideally, get used to doing without, it's much better for you.

Vegetarian variety

Don't worry if you're vegetarian, you can have all the meals I suggest, but substitute vegetarian equivalents for the meat, e.g. lasagne made with Quorn, or a chop suey made with tofu. You can either buy ready-made or make your own, using the recipes at the back of this book. For sandwich fillings, use vegetarian equivalents – you can buy vegetarian 'ham', 'bacon' and pâté, for example, as well as vegetarian cheese.

Star tips for success

Don't let yourself feel hungry. If you do get hunger pangs, drink a glass of sparkling mineral water or a diet sparkling drink to take the edge off your appetite. Alternatively, chew a piece of sugar-free gum or suck a sugar-free sweet (but be careful, some sweets are high in sorbitol, which can upset your stomach if you have too much). If necessary, bring your meal forward slightly so you eat before you get too hungry. If you are desperate, have one of your snack allowances, but don't gobble it, eat it slowly and enjoy it. See also the tips in Chapter 2.

Chapter 6
Your 28-day Diet Plan

This section contains your complete, balanced diet plan for four whole weeks. No counting, no planning – just follow the daily diets as they are listed. Each day's plan is complete in itself, so you must not swap meals from different days. Not only will the calorie counts not work but also the balance of nutrients will be wrong. However, you can swap whole days – the order of days is not important. You can, of course, have your main meal at lunchtime and the lunch menu in the evening if that suits your lifestyle better. You can use ready-made meals or the home-made options in the recipes at the back of the book. If you buy convenience foods, read the labels and buy low-fat options wherever possible.

All portions are average. Use your common sense here: an 'average' steak or fillet of fish is approximately 175 g/6 oz. If you are buying a ready-made dish designed for four portions, your average portion will be a quarter of the dish. The same applies to the recipes at the back of the book, which are all made to serve four.

Where there is no stated quantity for vegetables, have as many as you like. Where quantities are given in spoonfuls, use a tablespoon of the type you use to serve your food at the table, level unless heaped is called for. Where small spoonfuls or teaspoonfuls are called for, use an ordinary teaspoon. There is no need to use proper measuring spoons.

You may drink as much water (sparkling or still), tea or coffee (black or with just a splash of skimmed milk) and 'diet' soft drinks as you wish, but I don't advise too much caffeine or carbonated drinks.

Key to symbols

✗ Denotes a made-up dish, such as lasagne, shepherd's pie, fish pie, etc. You can either buy these ready-made, or use the recipes at the back of the book. The page references are given in brackets.

♦ Denotes additional items **for men only**. In most cases, these are simply larger portions to be substituted for the quantity in the meal plan – for example, on Day 1, men are allowed **three** sausages for dinner instead of two. In a few cases, men are given an additional item not included in the normal meal plan, such as jam (conserve) on their toast, or a banana.

Day 1

Breakfast

A small glass of pure fruit juice

A bowl of corn flakes with skimmed milk

Lunch

1 round of tuna and cucumber sandwiches, made with 2 slices
of medium-sliced bread, with a scraping of low-fat spread and
⅓ standard can of tuna in brine, not oil

An apple

Dinner

2 (♀ 3) extra-lean thick sausages, grilled (broiled)
3 (♀ 7) heaped spoonfuls of mashed potatoes
Broccoli and carrots
Thin gravy

A small bowl of stewed rhubarb OR 2 canned pear halves in
natural juice
2 spoonfuls of low-fat canned custard

Day 2

Breakfast

A small glass of pure fruit juice

1 (✝ 2) slice(s) of toast with a scraping of low-fat spread and
  grilled (broiled) or canned tomatoes

Lunch

Low-calorie pasta salad (✗ see page 121)

A pear

Dinner

Chicken and vegetable stir-fry (✗ see page 110)

2 scoops of low-calorie ice cream

✝ **For men only**

Day 3

Breakfast
A small glass of pure fruit juice

1 (♀ 2) Shredded Wheat with skimmed milk

Lunch
1 slice of cheese on toast, made with low-fat Cheddar cheese
A mixed salad OR 1 standard hamburger in a bun with salad

1 carton of low-calorie flavoured yoghurt

Dinner
1 fillet of poached smoked haddock on a bed of spinach
Canned or stewed tomatoes
5 (♀ 9) small new potatoes

1 large wedge of melon with a sprinkling of ground ginger
(optional)

Day 4

Breakfast

A small glass of pure fruit juice

2 (♀ 4) oat cakes with a scraping of low-fat spread and reduced-sugar jam (conserve) or marmalade

Lunch

Cheese and coleslaw wrap, made with a good handful of grated low-fat cheese, a good spoonful of low-calorie coleslaw and 1 flour tortilla

An apple

Dinner

Grilled (broiled) lean gammon steak with 1 slice of pineapple in natural juice

3 heaped spoonfuls of peas

3 (♀ 7) small new potatoes

1 carton of low-calorie flavoured yoghurt

Day 5

Breakfast

6 prunes in natural juice with 3 spoonfuls of plain low-fat yoghurt

1 (♀ 3) rye crispbread(s) with a scraping of low-fat spread and Marmite or reduced-sugar jam (conserve)

Lunch

Ham and tomato omelette, made with 2 eggs (roll it up, cold, for a packed lunch)

1 medium slice of focaccia bread

A pear

Dinner

1 grilled (broiled) salmon steak

A large mixed salad with any low-calorie dressing (✕ see pages 159–63)

1 small pot of low-fat fromage frais

Day 6

Breakfast
A small glass of pure fruit juice

1 boiled egg
1 (♀ 2) slice(s) of toast with a scraping of low-fat spread

Lunch
1 round of Marmite and salad sandwiches, made with 2 slices of
    medium-sliced bread and a scraping of low-fat spread

A satsuma or clementine

Dinner
Cauliflower cheese with tomatoes (✗ see page 140), served
    with a small can of tomatoes if using ready-made cauliflower
    cheese
2 slices of garlic bread

1 banana
1 scoop of low-calorie ice cream

Day 7

Breakfast
A small glass of pure fruit juice

1 (♈ 2) slice(s) of toast with a scraping of low-fat spread and grilled (broiled) or stewed mushrooms

Lunch
Chicken noodle soup
1 bread roll

An apple

Dinner
3 slices of lean roast lamb
A spoonful of mint sauce
Gravy
2 (♈ 4) pieces of roast potato
Carrots
Spring (collard) greens

A bowl of fresh fruit salad in natural juice
1 spoonful of low-fat crème fraîche

Day 8

Breakfast

½ grapefruit OR a small glass of pure juice

1 (♥ 2) crumpet(s) with a scraping of low-fat spread and reduced-sugar jam (conserve) or marmalade

Lunch

1 pitta bread, filled with 2 slices of pressed chicken roll and salad with a teaspoon of low-calorie mayonnaise

1 carton of low-calorie flavoured yoghurt

Dinner

Chilli con carne (✗ see page 120)

2 (♥ 4) spoonfuls of plain boiled rice

A green salad with any low-calorie dressing (✗ see pages 159–163)

Sugar-free fruit jelly (jello) OR a clementine or satsuma

Day 9

Breakfast

A small glass of pure fruit juice

1 rasher (slice) of lean grilled (broiled) back bacon
1 (♀ 2) poached egg(s)
½ grilled tomato
2 large grilled or stewed mushrooms
1 slice of toast with a scraping of low-fat spread

Lunch

1 prawn and salad roll, made with a scraping of low-fat spread, a heaped spoonful of prawns, your choice of salad and a teaspoon of low-calorie mayonnaise

A clementine or satsuma

Dinner

1 portion of lasagne (✗ see page 118)
A green salad with any low-calorie dressing (✗ see pages 159–163)

A bowl of fresh or thawed frozen raspberries

Day 10

Breakfast
A small glass of pure fruit juice

1 (♥ 2) toasted teacake(s) with a scraping of low-fat spread

Lunch
Vegetable soup (✗ see page 108)
1 (♥ 2) bread roll(s) with a scraping of low-fat spread

An apple

Dinner
Individual chicken and mushroom pie (✗ see page 122)
French (green) beans
Carrots OR turnips

A bowl of fresh or thawed frozen strawberries
1 spoonful of low-fat crème fraîche

♥ **For men only**

Day 11

Breakfast

A small glass of pure juice

A bowl of porridge with skimmed milk and half a teaspoon of sugar OR as much artificial sweetener as you like

Lunch

1 bread roll, filled with 2 spoonfuls of low-fat soft cheese mixed with cucumber and black pepper

A clementine or satsuma

Dinner

2 (♥ 4) grilled (broiled) fish cakes (✘ see page 128)
Grilled tomatoes
3 heaped spoonfuls of peas

1 canned pear half in natural juice
1 scoop of low-calorie chocolate ice cream, or other flavour of your choice

Day 12

Breakfast
A small glass of pure fruit juice

1 grilled (broiled) or jugged kipper
1 (👤 2) slice(s) of brown bread with a scraping of low-fat spread

Lunch
A mug of Marmite, Bovril or clear soup (canned or using stock
   powder)
2 (👤 4) rye crispbreads with a thin spreading of peanut butter
   and watercress

An apple

Dinner
1 grilled lean pork chop
Spaghetti with tomato and basil sauce (✗ see page 126)
A green salad with a little low-calorie dressing (✗ see pages
   159–163)

1 fresh fig OR a clementine or satsuma

Day 13

Breakfast

A small glass of pure fruit juice

A bowl of corn flakes with skimmed milk
♱ 1 sliced banana

Lunch

1 round of egg and cress sandwiches, made with 2 slices of medium-sliced bread, 1 hard-boiled (hard-cooked) egg and a scraping of low-fat spread

10 fresh cherries OR a kiwi fruit

Dinner

1 grilled (broiled) turkey breast steak
1 spoonful of cranberry sauce
3 (♱ 5) spoonfuls of mashed potatoes
Mangetout

1 carton of low-calorie flavoured yoghurt

♱ For men only

Day 14

Breakfast

A small glass of pure fruit juice

1 (♦ 2) slice(s) of toast with a scraping of low-fat spread and grilled (broiled) or stewed mushrooms

Lunch

Tomato and orange soup (✗ see page 106)

2 (♦ 4) rye crispbreads with a scraping of low-fat spread and Marmite

1 large plum

Dinner

4 thin slices of roast beef
Gravy
1 spoonful of horseradish relish
1 Yorkshire pudding
2 (♦ 4) pieces of roast potato
Carrots
Broccoli

Sugar-free jelly (jello) with fruit, fresh, chopped or canned in natural juice

Day 15

Breakfast
A small glass of pure fruit juice

1 (**♦** 2) toasted English muffin(s) with a scraping of low-fat spread and reduced-sugar jam (conserve) or marmalade

Lunch
1 round of salmon and cucumber sandwiches, made with 2 slices of medium-sliced bread, a scraping of low-fat spread and ⅓ standard can of salmon

A pear

Dinner
3 thin slices of cold roast beef
3 (**♦** 5) spoonfuls of mashed potatoes
A large mixed salad with any low-calorie dressing (**✗** see pages 159–163)

1 carton of low-calorie flavoured yoghurt

Day 16

Breakfast

A small glass of pure fruit juice

1 slice of toast, spread with a spoonful of low-fat soft cheese and
a pinch of ground cinnamon, topped with 1 banana, sliced

Lunch

4 crab sticks
A mixed salad
1 small spoonful of low-calorie mayonnaise

1 carton of low-calorie flavoured yoghurt

Dinner

Beef chow mein (✗ see page 112)

2 slices of pineapple, fresh, or canned in natural juice

Day 17

Breakfast

A small glass of pure fruit juice

A bowl of branflakes, with skimmed milk

Lunch

1 bread roll with a scraping of low-fat spread plus filling: 2 slices of bresaola OR 1 slice of lean ham; 1 sliced tomato and a little chopped, fresh basil

1 carton of low-fat fromage frais

Dinner

Veal or pork escalope in breadcrumbs, grilled (broiled) or baked
A wedge of lemon
3 (🕴 5) heaped spoonfuls of mashed potatoes
French (green) beans

5 apricot halves, canned in natural juice

Day 18

Breakfast
A large wedge of melon

1 (✝ 2) slice(s) of toast, with a scraping of low-fat spread and reduced-sugar jam (conserve) or marmalade

Lunch
1 jacket potato, topped with a small handful of grated reduced-fat Cheddar or Dutch cheese
✝ 1 small can of reduced-sugar baked beans in tomato sauce

An apple

Dinner
2 chicken fajitas (✗ see page 114)
A large mixed salad with any low-calorie dressing (✗ see pages 159–163)

1 carton of plain low-fat yoghurt with a teaspoonful of clear honey

✝ **For men only**

Day 19

Breakfast

A small glass of pure fruit juice

1 scrambled egg
1 (♥ 2) slice(s) of toast with a scraping of low-fat spread

Lunch

A mug of Marmite, Bovril or clear soup
2 rice cakes, each topped with a spoonful of low-fat cheese
  spread
4 cherry tomatoes

A banana

Dinner

Cod with parsley sauce (✗ see page 155)
3 (♥ 6) pieces of plain boiled potatoes
3 spoonfuls of mixed peas and sweetcorn (corn)

A clementine or satsuma

Day 20

Breakfast
A small glass of pure fruit juice

1 (♀ 2) rashers (slices) of grilled (broiled) lean back bacon
1 grilled tomato
1 (♀ 2) rye crispbread(s) with a scraping of low-fat spread

Lunch
2 hard-boiled (hard-cooked) eggs
A mixed salad
A spoonful of low-calorie mayonnaise

1 carton of low-calorie flavoured yoghurt

Dinner
Irish stew (✗ see page 136)

½ fresh mango OR mandarin oranges, canned in natural juice

Day 21

Breakfast

A small glass of pure fruit juice

A bowl of corn flakes with skimmed milk

Lunch

1 small (♦ 2 or 1 large) can(s) of reduced-sugar baked beans in tomato sauce
1 (♦ 2) slice(s) of toast with a scraping of low-fat spread

1 large plum

Dinner

3 slices of skinless roast chicken
1 spoonful of stuffing
Gravy
2 (♦ 4) pieces of roast potato
Cauliflower
Mangetout

5 lychees, fresh or canned in natural juice

Day 22

Breakfast
A small glass of pure fruit juice

1 (♀ 2) slice(s) of toast with a scraping of low-fat spread and grilled (broiled) or stewed mushrooms
♀ A scraping of reduced-sugar jam (conserve) or marmalade on the second slice of toast

Lunch
1 wholemeal pitta bread, filled with 1 small carton of plain or flavoured low-fat cottage cheese and salad

An apple

Dinner
Spaghetti carbonara (✗ see page 127)
A green salad with any low-calorie dressing (✗ see pages 159–163)

1 canned peach half in natural juice, drained
1 scoop of low-calorie ice cream

Day 23

Breakfast
A small glass of pure fruit juice

1 (✝ 2) Weetabix with skimmed milk
✝ 1 banana OR a good handful of raisins

Lunch
1 hot dog in a bun with onions

An apple

Dinner
Cottage pie (✗ see page 124)
Cabbage
Carrots

1 carton of low-fat fromage frais

✝ For men only

Day 24

Breakfast
A small glass of pure fruit juice

2 (♥ 4) oat cakes with a scraping of low-fat spread and reduced-sugar jam (conserve) or marmalade

Lunch
Carrot and coriander soup (✗ see page 104)
1 (♥ 2) bread roll(s)

A clementine or satsuma

Dinner
1 large slice of quiche Lorraine (✗ see page 142)
A large mixed salad with any low-calorie dressing (✗ see pages 159–163)

A small bowl of stewed blackberries and apple
1 spoonful of low-fat crème fraîche

Day 25

Breakfast
A small glass of pure fruit juice
1 slice of toast with a scraping of low-fat spread and grilled (broiled) or canned tomatoes

Lunch
2 (♥ 3) crispy taco shells, filled with salad and a small handful of grated reduced-fat Cheddar or Dutch cheese

A small orange

Dinner
Fish pie, topped with potato (✗ see page 130)
Carrots
Mangetout

1 scoop of low-calorie ice cream

Day 26

Breakfast

A small glass of pure fruit juice

A bowl of corn flakes with skimmed milk

Lunch

1 (♟ 2) slice(s) of toast with a scraping of low-fat spread and 3 (♟ 6) sardines

A small bunch of grapes

Dinner

Sweet and sour chicken, not in batter (✗ see page 113)

½ block of Chinese egg noodles

A large beansprout and cucumber salad, sprinkled with soy sauce and lemon juice or soy dressing (✗ see page 160)

2 slices of pineapple, fresh or canned in natural juice

Day 27

Breakfast
½ grapefruit

1 (♦ 2) crumpet(s) with a scraping of low-fat spread and clear honey

Lunch
Leek and potato soup (✗ see page 105)
1 thick slice of crusty bread

10 cherries OR a clementine or satsuma

Dinner
1 lean pork chop, brushed with bottled barbecue sauce and grilled (broiled)
6 (♦ 9) potato wedges, grilled (broiled) or baked
Broccoli and cauliflower OR a large mixed salad with any low-calorie dressing (✗ see pages 159–163)

1 carton of low-calorie flavoured yoghurt

Day 28

Breakfast
A small glass of pure fruit juice

A bowl of Sultana Bran or branflakes with skimmed milk

Lunch
2 (♀ 4) rye crispbreads
1 (♀ 2) individual Baby Bel cheese(s)
1 tomato
Slices of cucumber, a spoonful of sweet pickle and 2 pickled
  onions

An apple

Dinner
2 thick slices of lean roast pork (without crackling!)
1 spoonful of apple sauce
1 spoonful of stuffing
Gravy
2 (♀ 4) pieces of roast potatoes
Broccoli
Carrots

1 scoop of lemon sorbet

Chapter 7
Special Occasions

Eating out and entertaining can be a real problem if you are on a diet. You don't want to bore all your friends with your efforts not to break your diet and you don't want to undo all the good you've worked so hard to achieve. However, with my diet plan, help is at hand.

As before, you must keep to a complete day's diet plan, so on page 96 you will find breakfast and lunch/supper ideas for the special day. Choose from these for your breakfast and ordinary lunch or supper that you need for the day.

If you going to a restaurant to eat, choose a meal from the restaurant menu that is made up of any of the options on pages 97–99 (or as close as you can get). To really treat yourself, save up snack points in the preceding days (as suggested on page 56) so that you can have a calorific pudding and/or some extra alcohol.

If you are entertaining at home, make up the meal from the 'special occasion' recipe selection on pages 164–88. Note that the puddings in that section can be eaten without having to save up any snack points, which should leave you more points to use on wine or after-dinner mints!

Diet plan for special-occasion days

Remember, you must have breakfast and a meal made up from the options here, in addition to your special occasion meal.

Breakfast
A small glass of pure fruit juice

2 (♥ 4) crispbreads with a scraping of low-fat spread and Marmite, reduced-sugar jam (conserve) or marmalade

Lunch or supper
1 hard-boiled (hard-cooked) egg
OR 4 slices of pressed chicken roll
OR 2 medium slices of lean ham
OR ½ standard can of tuna in brine, drained
A large mixed salad
1 spoonful of any low-calorie dressing (✗ see pages 159–163)
♥ 1 bread roll with a scraping of low-fat spread

A satsuma or clementine

Restaurant meals

It is perfectly possible to eat out without ruining your diet. When you come to look at the menu, follow these simple rules.

Avoid nuts, pâtés, avocados, puff pastry (paste), salamis and other sausages, pancakes and pizzas (I know we have said one slice is okay, but when you're out, you'll have a whole one, which is highly calorific).

Any kind of food cooked in loads of oil or butter is absolutely forbidden, including chips (fries) and other deep-fried foods, e.g. scampi or squid, in batter or breadcrumbs.

Also keep away from anything flambéed and anything presented with a cream sauce, whether it's hot or cold.

Choose from the following, if possible, or the nearest you can get. If none of these is available, use your common sense and go for options with the lowest calorie counts. If your choice comes bathed in butter, oil or vinaigrette, leave as much as you can bear!

Starters
Asparagus
Carpaccio (wafer-thin slices) of beef
Florida cocktail
Fresh seafood platter
Garlic bread – 2 slices only
Globe artichoke
Grilled (broiled) grapefruit
Melon cocktail

Moules à la marinière
Oysters
Parma ham and melon
Roasted Mediterranean vegetables
Salad options – ask for just a little dressing
Smoked salmon
Thin soup – not creamed

Main courses
Any grilled (broiled) or poached meat, poultry or fish
Byriani dishes
Casseroles, e.g. boeuf bourguignon, coq au vin, chicken marengo,
    beef in beer, etc. – avoid those laced with cream or butter
Chilli con carne
Chinese stir-fries, e.g. chop suey and chow mein
Kebabs
Pasta or rice dish e.g. lasagne, risotto or paella – not those
    bathed in cream or thick sauces
Salad options (see Starters, above)
Tandoori meat or chicken
Vegetable curry – not meat or poultry curries, as these tend to be
    highly calorific

Side dishes
Green, yellow and red vegetables, steamed or boiled: Eat as
many as you like.

Salad: Eat as much as you like. You can have just a tiny spoonful of ordinary dressing but if low-calorie is available, have a good spoonful. If oil and vinegar are offered, have just the tiniest drizzle of oil (or, preferably, none at all), then vinegar to taste.

Potatoes: Choose jacket, new or Duchesse. Avoid chips (fries) or speciality potato dishes, such as Dauphinoise. Do not add butter or dressing of any kind.

Plain rice, pasta or couscous: Have only a small serving.

Desserts
You should, with any luck, have saved up enough points to have a calorific dessert. Most of the acceptable choices are listed in the snacks starting on page 57, so you'll know what you can go for. If not, choose fresh fruit salad or a fruit sorbet. Avoid added cream.

Chapter 8
Maintaining the New You

So you've reached your ideal weight – congratulations! By now you should have got used to your new way of eating: you're allowing yourself snacks only when you really want them; you eat at least five portions of fruit and vegetables a day and you make sure you don't let yourself feel hungry. You should also, hopefully, be enjoying your food, looking forward to meals and savouring every mouthful.

The challenge now is to keep your weight down. The solution is straightforward – you must have no more calories than you burn up every day, eat a healthy diet and exercise regularly. Remember, though, that you don't want too few calories either. Women need approximately 1,900 calories to maintain a healthy weight. Up until now you have been having around 1,200 (if you've had your quota of snacks). Men need, on average, around 2,300 calories per day.

Every day you need to have similar meals to those you ate while on the diet. You can, of course, eat other things as long as you bear in mind the tips I gave you in Chapters 2, 3 and 4. You also need to increase your complex carbohydrate levels to maintain your new weight.

- Eat as before but add up to four extra slices of bread a day plus an extra portion of rice, pasta, couscous, bulghar (cracked wheat), potatoes, yams or sweet potatoes. From time to time you can also have parsnips, plantains or breadfruit, and the odd avocado or handful of nuts.
- Do not increase your fat levels. Ideally, stick to low-fat spreads and dairy products. You can, however, have semi-skimmed milk instead of skimmed if you prefer and use a little olive or sunflower oil in dressings and for cooking.
- Keep taking regular exercise.

You should also stick to the 6-point snack system, trying to choose snacks from the 1-point list whenever possible. You can relax it a bit, but if you have, say, 12 points-worth of snacks one day, have none – or very few – the next. You can also allow yourself an occasional really calorie-laden treat, such as a Danish pastry or a full-size chocolate bar. But you must remember to keep your snack levels well down the following day. It's purely a case of long-term management.

Finding your benchmark

Weigh yourself one week after going on the maintenance diet. If you are gaining weight, halve the extras you are eating. Check again a week later and readjust if necessary. Once your weight is stable, that's the level of calories you need from now on.

Chapter 9
Everyday Diet Plan Recipes

This chapter contains all the recipes used in the diet plan. But, you don't have to cook if you don't want to; you can buy ready-made options instead. Look for low-fat packs (obviously, the lower the calories and fat, the better) and choose whichever brands you prefer.

All these recipes have suggestions for accompaniments included in the diet plan.

I have also given a large number of everyday recipes that can be used when you've finished the reducing diet plan but want to maintain a healthy diet and weight. They are all low in fat and calories to give you really nutritious meals. Serve the main courses with a green salad, dressed with lemon juice and black pepper or a little low-calorie dressing, or with any steamed or boiled green or root vegetables of your choice.

Notes on the Recipes

- Measures are given in metric, imperial and American units. Follow one set only – do not mix.
- American terms are given in brackets.
- All spoon measurements are level: 1 tsp = 5 ml, 1 tbsp = 15 ml.
- Eggs are medium unless otherwise stated.
- Always wash, peel, core and seed, if necessary, fresh produce before use.
- Always use fresh herbs unless dried are specifically called for. If you have to substitute dried for fresh, use half the quantity stated. When garnishing, there is no substitute for sprigs of fresh parsley or coriander (cilantro).
- Seasoning and the use of strongly flavoured ingredients, such as onions and garlic, are very much a matter of personal preference. Test the food as you cook and adjust to suit your taste.
- Can and packet sizes are approximate and will depend on the particular brand.
- Where low-fat spread is called for, use the brand of your choice, but check the label to make sure that it is suitable for cooking.

Soups

Soups make filling starters, which will help you to avoid calorific main courses and desserts, and are especially welcome in cold weather. You can make them in large quantities and freeze them in small batches to eat as and when you want them.

Carrot and Coriander Soup

Serves 4

450 g/1 lb carrots, chopped
1 onion, chopped
750 ml/1¼ pts/5 cups vegetable stock, made with 2 stock cubes
2.5 ml/½ tsp ground coriander (cilantro)
2.5 ml/½ tsp ground cumin
A pinch of grated nutmeg
2.5 ml/½ tsp dried mixed herbs
Freshly ground black pepper
15 ml/1 tbsp chopped fresh coriander

1 Put the carrots, onion and stock in a saucepan with the spices and herbs. Add plenty of pepper and bring to the boil. Reduce the heat, part-cover and simmer for 30 minutes.
2 Purée the soup in a blender or food processor, then return to the saucepan. Reheat, season with a little more pepper, if liked, and serve garnished with chopped coriander.

Leek and Potato Soup
Serves 4–6

15 g/¹/₂ oz/1 tbsp low-fat spread
2 large leeks, sliced
1 onion, roughly chopped
1 large potato, peeled and diced
1 bouquet garni sachet
600 ml/1 pt/2¹/₂ cups vegetable stock, made with 1 stock cube
Salt and freshly ground black pepper
300 ml/¹/₂ pt/1¹/₄ cups skimmed milk
15 ml/1 tbsp chopped fresh parsley

1 Heat the spread in a saucepan. Add the leeks and onion and fry (sauté), stirring, for 2 minutes until softened but not browned. Add the potato and cook for 1 minute, stirring.
2 Add the bouquet garni and stock and a little salt and pepper. Bring to the boil, reduce the heat, part-cover and simmer gently for 15–20 minutes until the vegetables are really soft.
3 Purée the soup in a blender or food processor and return to the pan. Stir in the milk and heat through. Taste and re-season if necessary.
4 Ladle into warm soup bowls and garnish with the chopped parsley. Alternatively, turn into a large bowl, leave until cold, then stir in the milk, re-season and chill until ready to serve in cold bowls, garnished with the parsley.

Tomato and Orange Soup
This is also delicious served chilled, topped with
chopped fresh basil instead of chives.

Serves 4

1 orange
150 ml/¼ pt/⅔ cup water
1 onion, roughly chopped
15 g/½ oz/1 tbsp low-fat spread
400 g/14 oz/1 large can of chopped tomatoes
300 ml/½ pt/1¼ cups vegetable stock, made with 1 stock cube
30 ml/2 tbsp tomato purée (paste)
Finely grated rind and juice of ½ lemon
5 ml/1 tsp caster (superfine) sugar
Salt and freshly ground black pepper
15 ml/1 tbsp snipped fresh chives

1 Thinly pare the rind from the orange and cut into thin strips. Squeeze the juice and reserve. Boil the rind in the water for 3 minutes. Lift the rind out of the water with a draining spoon and leave to cool. Reserve the cooking water.
2 Meanwhile, in a separate pan, fry (sauté) the onion in the spread for 2 minutes, stirring, until softened but not browned.
3 Add the orange cooking water, orange juice and all the remaining ingredients except the chives. Bring to the boil and simmer for 5 minutes. Turn into a blender or food processor and purée until smooth.

4 Return to the pan, season to taste and reheat. Ladle into warm soup bowls, garnish with the reserved orange rind and chives and serve straight away.

Chilled Cucumber and Mint Soup

Change the flavour, if you like, by using dried dill (dill weed) instead of mint, and white wine vinegar instead of the cider vinegar. Note that this soup does not freeze well.

Serves 4

1 cucumber
Salt
10 ml/2 tsp dried mint
30 ml/2 tbsp cider vinegar
Freshly ground black pepper
300 ml/½ pt/1¼ cups plain low-fat yoghurt
300 ml/½ pt/1¼ cups skimmed milk

1 Cut four thin slices off the cucumber and reserve for garnish.
2 Coarsely grate the remainder into a bowl. Sprinkle with salt and leave to stand for 10 minutes to draw out the moisture. Squeeze out all the moisture and drain off.
3 Stir in the mint, vinegar, a good grinding of pepper and then stir in the yoghurt. Chill for at least 1 hour.
4 When ready to serve, stir in the milk, ladle into soup bowls and float a slice of cucumber on each.

Vegetable Soup

*You can make this with a mixture of frozen peas, diced carrot,
swede (rutabaga), turnip and potato instead of the
frozen mixed vegetables, if you like.*

Serves 4

15 g/½ oz/1 tbsp low-fat spread
1 onion, finely chopped
450 g/1 lb frozen diced mixed vegetables
450 ml/¾ pt/2 cups vegetable stock, made with 1 stock cube
1 bay leaf
Salt and freshly ground black pepper
15 ml/1 tbsp cornflour (cornstarch)
600 ml/1 pt/2½ cups passata (sieved tomatoes)

1 Heat the spread in a large saucepan. Add the onion and fry
  (sauté) for 2 minutes, stirring until softened but not browned.
2 Add the frozen vegetables, stock, bay leaf and seasoning.
  Bring to the boil, part-cover, reduce the heat and simmer for
  15 minutes until really tender.
3 Blend the cornflour with a little of the passata. Stir in the
  remaining passata. Add to the pan, bring to the boil and cook
  for 2 minutes, stirring until slightly thickened.
4 Taste and adjust the seasoning. Remove the bay leaf and serve
  hot.

Russian Beetroot Soup

*For an alternative refreshing starter or lunch, prepare the
vegetables in the same way, mix with the crème fraîche, season
with salt, pepper, the dill (dill weed) and a dash of vinegar,
then spoon on to crisp lettuce leaves.*

Serves 6

2 carrots
1 onion
4 cooked beetroot (red beets)
2 celery sticks
900 ml/1½ pts/3¾ cups beef or vegetable stock, made with
    2 stock cubes
15 ml/1 tbsp red wine vinegar
2.5 ml/½ tsp dried dill
Salt and freshly ground black pepper
20 ml/4 tsp low-fat crème fraîche
15 ml/1 tbsp snipped fresh chives

1 Grate the carrots, onion, beetroot and celery (discard the
  strings) and place in a saucepan. Add the stock, vinegar and
  dill and bring to the boil. Reduce the heat, cover and simmer
  gently for 20 minutes until the vegetables are tender.
2 Season to taste. Ladle into warm soup bowls and put a
  spoonful of crème fraîche on top. Sprinkle with the chives
  and serve. Alternatively, put the soup in a large bowl to cool,
  then chill before garnishing and serving.

Main Courses

You don't always want to eat bought ready-prepared meals, but if you use ordinary recipe books for home-made dishes, you can't be sure that you are making a low-calorie version. All the dishes in this section are calorie-counted and provide an excellent recipe bank for your new healthy eating maintenance plan.

Chicken and Vegetable Stir-fry

Ring the changes by using some other vegetables for this, such as strips of courgette (zucchini), cucumber, celeriac (celery root) or baby corn cobs, cut into two or three pieces, or shredded pak choi or French (green) beans, cut into short lengths. Bear in mind colour and texture when making your choices.

Serves 4

175 g/6 oz/³/₄ cup long-grain rice
25 g/1 oz/2 tbsp low-fat spread
225 g/8 oz chicken stir-fry meat
1 bunch of spring onions (scallions), cut into short lengths
1 red and 1 green (bell) pepper, cut into thin strips
1 carrot, cut into thin matchsticks
¼ small green cabbage, cut into thin shreds
100 g/4 oz button mushrooms, sliced
225 g/8 oz/4 cups beansprouts
150 ml/¼ pt/²/₃ cup chicken stock, made with ½ stock cube
15 ml/1 tbsp soy sauce
2.5 ml/½ tsp ground ginger

1 Cook the rice according to the packet directions. Drain.
2 Meanwhile, heat the oil in a large non-stick frying pan (skillet) or wok. Add the chicken, spring onions, peppers and carrot and stir-fry for 4 minutes.
3 Add the cabbage, mushrooms and beansprouts and stir-fry for a further 2 minutes. Add the stock, soy sauce and ginger and bring to the boil. Reduce the heat, cover with a lid and cook for 2 minutes.
4 Spoon the rice into warm bowls. Pile the chicken stir-fry on top and serve.

Beef Chow Mein

Serves 4

100 g/4 oz quick-cook Chinese egg noodles
2 onions, halved and cut into wedges
15 ml/1 tbsp sunflower oil
225 g/8 oz beef stir-fry meat or fillet steak, cut into thin strips
1 carrot, cut into thin matchsticks
1 courgette (zucchini), cut into thin matchsticks
1 green (bell) pepper, cut into thin strips
3 tomatoes, cut into wedges
100 g/4 oz button mushrooms, sliced
30 ml/2 tbsp sherry
2.5 ml/½ tsp Chinese five-spice powder
45 ml/3 tbsp soy sauce
15 ml/1 tbsp clear honey

1 Cook the noodles according to the packet directions, then drain and reserve.
2 Separate the onion wedges into layers. Heat the oil in a large non-stick frying pan (skillet) or wok. Stir-fry the onions and steak for 2 minutes.
3 Add the carrot and courgette and stir-fry for a further 3 minutes.
4 Add the remaining ingredients and cook, stirring, for 5 minutes.
5 Stir in the noodles and cook for a further minute. Serve straight away.

Sweet and Sour Chicken

*For a tasty alternative, use pork fillet instead of the chicken and
add a crushed garlic clove with the spring onions (scallions).*

Serves 4

¹/₄ cucumber, chopped
2 spring onions, chopped
225 g/8 oz/1 small can of chopped tomatoes
225 g/8 oz/1 small can of pineapple chunks in natural juice
450 g/1 lb chicken breast fillets, cut into dice
20 ml/1¹/₂ tbsp cornflour (cornstarch)
30 ml/2 tbsp soy sauce
A good pinch of caster (superfine) sugar (optional)
Plain boiled rice, to serve

1 Put the cucumber, spring onions, chopped tomatoes and the
  can of pineapple with its juice in a saucepan. Bring to the boil
  and simmer for 3 minutes.
2 Add the chicken and simmer for a further 6 minutes until the
  chicken is tender. Blend the cornflour with the soy sauce and
  stir into the mixture. Bring to the boil and cook for 2 minutes,
  stirring gently. Taste and add a little caster sugar, if liked.
3 Spoon on to a bed of boiled rice and serve.

Chicken Fajitas

*For a change, try serving the chicken breasts on top of the
cooked vegetables, garnished with the crème fraîche and
shredded lettuce, with a portion of noodles or rice on the side
(omit the flour tortillas, of course).*

Serves 4

4 skinless chicken breasts
1 large garlic clove, crushed
Finely grated rind and juice of 1 lime
1 red chilli, seeded and finely chopped
15 ml/1 tbsp paprika
5 ml/1 tsp dried oregano
2.5 ml/½ tsp ground cumin
1.5 ml/¼ tsp ground cinnamon
40 g/1½ oz/3 tbsp low-fat spread, melted
Salt and freshly ground black pepper
1 red (bell) pepper, cut into 8 thick strips
1 green pepper, cut into 8 thick strips
1 aubergine (eggplant), sliced
1 courgette (zucchini), cut diagonally into slices
8 flour tortillas
A small bowl of tomato or chilli relish
150 ml/¼ pt/⅔ cup low-fat crème fraîche
1 onion, finely chopped
1 small bowl of iceberg lettuce, finely shredded

1 Wipe the chicken breasts and slash in several places with a sharp knife. Place in a shallow dish. Mix together the garlic, lime rind and juice, chilli, paprika, oregano, cumin and cinnamon with half the melted spread. Season lightly with salt and pepper and pour over the chicken. Turn to coat completely. Cover and leave to marinate for at least 1 hour.

2 Lay the peppers, aubergine and courgette on a large sheet of foil, shiny side up. Drizzle with the rest of the melted spread and season with salt and pepper. Wrap up the parcel and twist the edges together to seal.

3 Place the parcel on a baking (cookie) sheet, positioning it to one side so there is room to add the chicken later, and bake in a preheated oven at 200°C/400°F/gas mark 6 (fan oven 180°C) for 15 minutes.

4 Add the chicken breasts to the baking sheet and cook for a further 15–20 minutes, turning the chicken once until cooked through. Wrap the tortillas in foil and put to warm on a low shelf in the oven for the last 5 minutes.

5 Remove everything from the oven. Cut the chicken into thin strips.

6 Arrange the chicken and vegetables on a warm plate. Serve with the stack of tortillas, the chilli relish, crème fraîche and the chopped onion and lettuce. Alternatively, divide the ingredients between the tortillas, roll up and serve.

Mixed Moussaka

*For a more traditional Greek-style moussaka, use
2 large aubergines (eggplants) and omit the potatoes and
courgettes (zucchini).*

Serves 4

2 potatoes, sliced
1 aubergine, sliced
2 courgettes, sliced
350 g/12 oz extra-lean minced (ground) beef
1 onion, chopped
1 garlic clove, crushed
5 ml/1 tsp ground cinnamon
2.5 ml/½ tsp dried marjoram
120 ml/4 fl oz/½ cup passata (sieved tomatoes)
30 ml/2 tbsp tomato purée (paste)
30 ml/2 tbsp chopped fresh parsley
Freshly ground black pepper
1 egg
150 ml/¼ pt/⅔ cup plain low-fat yoghurt
30 ml/2 tbsp grated strong low-fat Cheddar cheese

1 Boil the potatoes in a fairly large pan of lightly salted water
for 3 minutes. Add the aubergine and courgettes and continue
to boil for about 3 minutes or until all the vegetables are
tender but still hold their shape. Drain.

2 Put the beef, onion and garlic in a pan and fry (sauté) until the meat is brown and all the grains are separate. Spoon off any fat, but leave the juices.

3 Stir in the cinnamon and marjoram, the passata and tomato purée. Bring to the boil, reduce the heat and simmer for 15 minutes. Stir in the parsley and a good grinding of pepper.

4 Layer the vegetables and meat in an ovenproof dish, finishing with a layer of vegetables.

5 Beat the egg and yoghurt together with a good grinding of pepper and pour over the mixture. Sprinkle with the cheese. Bake in a preheated oven at 190°C/375°F/gas mark 5 (fan oven 170°C) for about 40 minutes until the top is set and golden brown.

Lasagne

If you want to make Spaghetti Bolognese instead, make the same meat mixture using steps 1 and 2 and serve it with plain boiled spaghetti and a sprinkling of freshly grated Parmesan cheese.

Serves 4

1 large onion, finely chopped
1 garlic clove, crushed
225 g/8 oz extra-lean minced (ground) beef
1 carrot, finely chopped
100 g/4 oz button mushrooms, sliced
400 g/14 oz/1 large can of chopped tomatoes
30 ml/2 tbsp red wine (optional)
15 ml/1 tbsp tomato purée (paste)
1 bay leaf
Salt and freshly ground black pepper
25 g/1 oz/¼ cup plain (all-purpose) flour
450 ml/¾ pt/2 cups skimmed milk
A small knob of low-fat spread
50 g/2 oz/½ cup reduced-fat Cheddar cheese, grated
8 sheets of no-need-to-precook lasagne

1 Put the onion, garlic, beef and carrot in a large non-stick saucepan. Cook, stirring, for 5 minutes until the meat is brown and all the grains are separate.

2 Add the mushrooms, tomatoes, wine, if using, the purée, bay leaf and seasoning to taste. Bring to the boil, stirring, then reduce the heat and simmer for 15 minutes, stirring occasionally, until the meat is bathed in a rich sauce.

3 Meanwhile, make the cheese sauce. Using a wire whisk, mix the flour with a little of the milk in a saucepan until smooth. Stir in the remaining milk and add the low-fat spread. Bring to the boil, stirring all the time with the whisk, and cook for 2 minutes. Season to taste and stir in half the cheese.

4 Spoon a little of the meat sauce into the base of a fairly shallow ovenproof dish. Top with a layer of lasagne, breaking it to fit. Continue to layer the meat and lasagne in this way, finishing with a layer of lasagne.

5 Spoon the cheese sauce over and sprinkle with the remaining cheese. Bake in a preheated oven at 190°C/375°F/gas mark 5 (fan oven 170°C) for 40 minutes until cooked through and golden on top.

Chilli Con Carne
Serves 4

To make delicious vegetarian chilli beans, omit the beef and add two more cans of kidney beans.

1 onion, finely chopped
225 g/8 oz extra-lean minced (ground) beef
1 garlic clove, crushed
2.5 ml/½ tsp chilli powder
5 ml/1 tsp ground cumin
5 ml/1 tsp dried oregano
400 g/14 oz/1 large can of chopped tomatoes
2 × 425 g/15 oz/2 large cans of red kidney beans, drained
15 ml/1 tbsp tomato purée (paste)
Salt and freshly ground black pepper

1 Put the onion, meat and garlic in a saucepan. Fry (sauté), stirring for 5 minutes until browned and all the grains of meat are separate. Spoon off any fat but leave the juices.
2 Stir in the spices and herbs and fry for 1 minute.
3 Add the tomatoes, kidney beans, tomato purée and salt and pepper. Bring to the boil, then reduce the heat and simmer for 30 minutes, stirring occasionally until the meat and beans are bathed in a rich sauce.
4 Taste and add more seasoning and chilli powder, if liked, before serving.

Low-calorie Pasta Salad

*If you don't like hot, spicy flavourings, use olive oil
instead of chilli oil.*

Serves 4

100 g/4 oz pasta shapes
200 g/7 oz/1 small can of naturally sweet sweetcorn (corn),
    drained
1 small green (bell) pepper, finely chopped
8 cherry tomatoes, quartered
5 cm/2 in piece of cucumber, diced
8 stuffed olives, sliced
15 ml/1 tbsp chilli oil
15 ml/1 tbsp water
15 ml/1 tbsp white wine vinegar
Salt and freshly ground black pepper
15 ml/1 tbsp chopped fresh coriander (cilantro)

1 Cook the pasta according to the packet directions. Drain,
  rinse with cold water and drain again. Turn into a salad bowl.
2 Add the sweetcorn, pepper, tomatoes, cucumber and olives.
3 Whisk the chilli oil and water together with the vinegar and a
  little salt and pepper. Pour over the salad and toss gently.
4 Spoon into individual bowls and sprinkle with the chopped
  coriander.

Individual Chicken and Mushroom Pies
*If you don't have shallow individual ovenproof dishes, this
quantity will fill a family-size pie dish.
The cooking time will be the same.*

Serves 4

225 g/8 oz/2 cups plain (all-purpose) flour
A good pinch of salt
100 g/4 oz/½ cup low-fat spread
A little cold water
225 g/8 oz chicken stir-fry meat
225 g/8 oz button mushrooms, sliced
5 ml/1 tsp dried minced (ground) onion
2.5 ml/½ tsp dried mixed herbs
295 g/10½ oz/1 medium can of condensed low-fat mushroom
    soup
Salt and freshly ground black pepper
A little skimmed milk, for glazing

1 Mix the flour and salt in a bowl. Add the spread and work
  with a fork until crumbly. Mix with enough cold water to
  form a soft but not sticky dough.
2 Knead gently on a lightly floured surface. Cut into four pieces
  and roll out each one to a circle slightly larger than the
  individual ovenproof dishes you are using.
3 Mix the chicken with the mushrooms, onion, herbs and soup.
  Season lightly and spoon into the dishes.

4 Roll out the pastry trimmings and cut into strips. Dampen the edges of the ovenproof dishes with water and press the strips on to the edges, then dampen these too.

5 Put the pastry rounds on top and press firmly round the edges. Press all round with the prongs of a fork to decorate and complete the seal. Make a small hole in the centre of each with a sharp knife to allow steam to escape.

6 Brush the pastry with the milk and bake in a preheated oven at 200°C/400°F/gas mark 6 (fan oven 180°C) for 15 minutes, then turn down the heat to 180°C/350°F/gas mark 4 (fan oven 160°C) for a further 20–25 minutes until golden and cooked through.

Cottage Pie

Make Shepherd's Pie instead, using lean minced (ground) lamb instead of beef. Alternatively, reduce the quantity of meat to 225 g/8 oz and give an interesting twist by adding a 425 g/15 oz/ large can of butter (lima) beans, drained before using.

Serves 4

1 onion, finely chopped
350 g/12 oz extra-lean minced beef
2 large carrots, finely chopped
75 g/3 oz frozen peas
¼ small green or white cabbage, finely shredded
450 ml/¾ pt/2 cups beef stock, made with 1 stock cube
A few drops of gravy browning
2.5 ml/½ tsp dried mixed herbs
Salt and freshly ground black pepper
700 g/1½ lb potatoes
30 ml/2 tbsp skimmed milk
10 g/¼ oz/2 tsp low-fat spread
25 g/1 oz/2 tbsp plain (all-purpose) flour

1 Put the onion, beef and carrots in a saucepan. Cook, stirring, for about 5 minutes until all the grains of meat are brown and separate. Spoon off any fat but leave the juices.

2 Add the peas, cabbage and stock. Stir in a few drops of gravy browning, the herbs and seasoning to taste. Part-cover and simmer very gently for 30 minutes or until tender and well flavoured.

3 Meanwhile, cut the potatoes into fairly small pieces and boil in lightly salted water until tender. Drain and mash well with the milk and low-fat spread.

4 Blend the flour with a little water and stir into the meat mixture. Bring back to the boil and cook for 2 minutes, stirring until thickened. Turn into a flameproof serving dish.

5 Top with the potato and fluff up with a fork. Brown under a preheated grill (broiler). Serve hot.

Spaghetti with Tomato and Basil Sauce

This is also good with 100 g/4 oz sliced mushrooms, stewed in a little water and added to the spaghetti after you have drained it.

Serves 4

225 g/8 oz spaghetti
300 ml/½ pt/1¼ cups passata (sieved tomatoes)
15 ml/1 tbsp tomato ketchup (catsup)
30 ml/2 tbsp chopped fresh basil
Salt and freshly ground black pepper
A few fresh basil leaves, for garnishing

1 Cook the spaghetti according to the packet directions. Drain and return to the saucepan.
2 Add the passata, ketchup and basil and season to taste. Toss over a gentle heat until hot through.
3 Serve straight away, garnished with a few extra basil leaves.

Spaghetti Carbonara

*If you don't like runny egg, you can cook the dish until the eggs
scramble, but the texture will not be so creamy or moist.*

Serves 4

225 g/8 oz spaghetti
50 g/2 oz pancetta or finely diced bacon (lardons)
1 onion, finely chopped
1 garlic clove, crushed
2 eggs, beaten
300 ml/½ pt/1¼ cups skimmed milk
30 ml/2 tbsp chopped fresh parsley
Salt and freshly ground black pepper

1 Cook the spaghetti according to the packet directions, drain
  and return to the saucepan.
2 Meanwhile, in a separate saucepan, cook the pancetta or
  diced bacon, onion and garlic, stirring over a gentle heat, until
  the the fat runs and the onion has softened. Cover with a lid
  and leave to 'sweat' over the lowest heat for about 10 minutes.
  Don't allow to brown too much. Tip into the cooked spaghetti.
3 Whisk the eggs with the milk and add to the pan. Add the
  parsley and some salt and lots of pepper. Cook, tossing and
  stirring, over a gentle heat until creamy. Don't cook too much
  or the sauce will scramble. Taste and add more seasoning if
  necessary.
4 Pile on to warm plates and serve.

Fish Cakes

Cod, haddock, whiting or any other chunky fish will make good fish cakes. These can be made up in advance, then chilled until you are ready to cook them.

Serves 4

2 potatoes, cut into fairly small chunks
225 g/8 oz white or smoked fish fillet, skinned
A small knob of low-fat spread
15 ml/1 tbsp chopped fresh parsley
5 ml/1 tsp curry powder
Salt and freshly ground black pepper
1 large egg, separated
45 ml/3 tbsp plain (all-purpose) flour
60 ml/4 tbsp dried breadcrumbs
15 ml/1 tbsp sunflower oil
Wedges of lemon and sprigs of fresh parsley, for garnishing

1 Put the potatoes in a pan, cover with cold water and add a pinch of salt.
2 Wrap the fish in foil, twisting and folding the edges to secure tightly.
3 Bring the potatoes to the boil, then add the foil parcel to the pan. Cover, reduce the heat slightly and cook for about 8 minutes or until the potatoes and fish are cooked through.

4 Lift out the foil parcel. Drain the potatoes and mash with the spread.

5 Unwrap the fish and flake with a fork. Add to the potato with the parsley, curry powder and some salt and pepper.

6 Beat the egg yolk and stir into the potato. Dust your hands with a little flour and shape the mixture into eight small, flat cakes.

7 Lightly whisk the egg white on a plate. Put the remaining flour and the breadcrumbs on two separate plates. Dip the cakes in the flour, then the egg white, then the breadcrumbs, to coat completely. Chill for at least 30 minutes.

8 When ready to serve, brush the surfaces of the cakes with the oil and grill (broil) for about 3 minutes on each side until golden and hot through. Garnish with wedges of lemon and sprigs of parsley and serve hot.

Fish Pie

This is also nice served in individual flameproof dishes. Try topping with crumbled reduced-fat Stilton cheese instead of the Cheddar for a change.

Serves 4

700 g/1½ lb potatoes, cut into bite-sized pieces
350 ml/12 fl oz/1⅓ cups skimmed milk
50 g/2 oz/½ cup strong reduced-fat Cheddar cheese, grated
100 g/4 oz button mushrooms, sliced
225 g/8 oz frozen mixed vegetables
1 bay leaf
450 g/1 lb white fish fillet
Salt and freshly ground black pepper
45 ml/3 tbsp plain (all-purpose) flour
30 ml/2 tbsp chopped fresh parsley

1 Cook the potatoes in boiling, lightly salted water until really tender. Drain and mash with 25 ml/1½ tbsp of the milk and half the cheese.

2 Meanwhile, put the mushrooms in a saucepan with the vegetables, bay leaf, fish and 300 ml/½ pt/1¼ cups of the remaining milk. Season to taste. Bring to the boil, then reduce the heat, part-cover and simmer gently for 8–10 minutes until the fish and vegetables are cooked.

3 Carefully, lift the fish out of the saucepan. Remove any skin and bones and roughly flake the flesh.

4 Blend the flour with the remaining milk until smooth. Stir into the vegetable mixture with the parsley. Bring to the boil and cook for 2 minutes, stirring until thickened. Discard the bay leaf.

5 Stir the fish into the sauce. Turn the mixture into a flameproof serving dish. Top with the cheesy potato and sprinkle with the remaining cheese. Grill (broil) for about 5 minutes until golden and piping hot. Serve straight away.

Smoked Salmon and Broccoli Tagliatelle

This is good made with 50 g/2 oz lean raw, cured ham, such as Parma ham, instead of the 100 g/4 oz smoked salmon.

Serves 4

225 g/8 oz tagliatelle
175 g/6 oz broccoli, cut into tiny florets
100 g/4 oz smoked salmon pieces, cut up if necessary
2 eggs
150 ml/¼ pt/⅔ cup low-fat crème fraîche
60 ml/4 tbsp skimmed milk
Salt and freshly ground black pepper
A squeeze of lemon juice
20 ml/4 tsp freshly grated Parmesan cheese

1 Cook the pasta according to the packet directions. Add the broccoli for the last 5 minutes of the cooking time. Drain and return to the saucepan.
2 Add the salmon and toss gently. Beat the eggs, crème fraîche and milk together and add to the pan with some salt and pepper.
3 Cook over a gentle heat, stirring until creamy but not totally scrambled. Taste and add lemon juice and a little more seasoning to taste.
4 Pile on to warm plates and sprinkle with the Parmesan cheese.

Cheesy-topped Prawn Bake
Serves 4

100 g/4 oz button mushrooms, sliced
1 large courgette (zucchini), thinly sliced
225 g/8 oz cooked peeled prawns (shrimp)
295 g/10½ oz/1 medium can of low-fat condensed mushroom
    soup
15 ml/1 tbsp tomato ketchup (catsup)
5 ml/1 tsp Worcestershire sauce
15 ml/1 tbsp chopped fresh parsley
50 g/2 oz/1 cup fresh breadcrumbs
100 g/4 oz/1 cup low-fat Cheddar cheese, grated
1 tomato, sliced
A few slices of cucumber

1 Put the mushrooms and courgette in a saucepan and add just enough water to cover. Bring to the boil, cover with a lid, then reduce the heat and simmer for 3 minutes. Drain and tip into an ovenproof serving dish.
2 Mix in the prawns, soup, ketchup, Worcestershire sauce, parsley, half the breadcrumbs and half the cheese.
3 Mix together the remaining breadcrumbs and cheese and sprinkle over. Bake in a preheated oven at 200°C/400°F/gas mark 6 (fan oven 180°C) for 25 minutes until golden.
4 Arrange the tomato and cucumber slices attractively on top and serve.

Salmon Parcels

You can use a 400 g/14 oz/large can of pink salmon instead of the salmon steaks for a very cheap, but still elegant, supper dish. Just drain the fish, remove the skin and bones if you prefer and separate into four portions.

Serves 4

4 sheets of filo pastry (paste)
15 ml/1 tbsp low-fat spread
4 small salmon steaks, about 150 g/5 oz each, skinned
4 mushrooms, finely chopped
2 tomatoes, finely chopped
Salt and freshly ground black pepper
5 ml/1 tsp dried basil
300 ml/½ pt/1¼ cups passata (sieved tomatoes)
Wedges of lemon and sprigs of fresh parsley, for garnishing

1 Lay the filo sheets on a work surface. Brush very lightly with a little of the spread, then fold each one in half.
2 Place a salmon steak on each folded piece and top with the mushrooms and tomatoes. Sprinkle with salt and pepper and half the basil. Wrap up the fish in the pastry and lay, sealed sides down, on a non-stick baking (cookie) sheet. Brush with the remaining spread.
3 Bake in a preheated oven at 200°C/400°F/gas mark 6 (fan oven 180°C) for 10–15 minutes until golden brown and the fish is cooked through.

4 Meanwhile, heat the passata in a small saucepan with the remaining basil and a little salt and pepper.
5 Spoon the passata on to warm plates. Top each with a salmon parcel, garnish with wedges of lemon and sprigs of parsley and serve.

Irish Stew

Irish stew is usually made with scrag end of lamb but this is rather fatty, so in this recipe I have used shoulder instead. You can cook the meat, leave to cool and then chill in the fridge overnight, ready to finish the dish the next day, if you prefer.

Serves 4

900 g/2 lb half-shoulder of lamb, trimmed of all fat and skin
2 large onions, quartered
1 bouquet garni sachet
Salt and freshly ground black pepper
3 large carrots, cut into chunks
2 large potatoes, quartered
30 ml/2 tbsp chopped fresh parsley

1 Put the lamb in a large saucepan with the onions, bouquet garni sachet and a little salt and pepper. Cover with water. Bring to the boil, reduce the heat, part-cover with a lid and simmer very gently for 1½ hours.
2 Leave to cool in the liquid. Skim the surface of all fat. Lift the lamb out and cut the meat into large chunks, discarding any remaining fat.
3 Return the meat to the pan. Add the prepared vegetables. Bring back to the boil, reduce the heat, part-cover and simmer gently for 30 minutes until the vegetables are really tender.
4 Ladle into warm bowls and sprinkle with chopped parsley before serving.

Tuna, Sweetcorn and Tomato Pasta Bake

*If you haven't got time to bake this, simply drain the cooked
pasta and return it to the pan. Add all the remaining ingredients
except the cheese and tomatoes and heat through in the
saucepan. Serve sprinkled with the cheese, with the sliced
tomatoes as a garnish.*

Serves 4

225 g/8 oz pasta shapes
185 g/6½ oz/1 standard can of tuna in brine, drained
200 g/7 oz/1 small can of naturally sweet sweetcorn (corn),
    drained
450 ml/¾ pt/2 cups passata (sieved tomatoes)
5 ml/1 tsp dried oregano
Freshly ground black pepper
50 g/2 oz/½ cup strong low-fat Cheddar cheese, grated
2 tomatoes, sliced

1 Cook the pasta in boiling, lightly salted water for 10 minutes
  or until just tender. Drain and turn into an ovenproof serving
  dish.
2 Add the tuna, sweetcorn, passata, oregano and lots of pepper
  and mix well.
3 Top with the cheese and arrange the tomato slices around the
  edge. Bake in a preheated oven at 190°C/375°F/gas mark 5
  (fan oven 170°C) for about 30 minutes until golden and
  bubbling.

Pork, Bamboo and Water Chestnut Stir-fry with Noodles

Serves 4

1 onion, halved and cut into chunky pieces
15 ml/1 tbsp sunflower oil
225 g/8 oz pork stir-fry meat
3 heads of pak choi, shredded
2 garlic cloves, finely chopped
225 g/8 oz/1 small can of water chestnuts, drained and sliced
225 g/8 oz/1 small can of bamboo shoots, drained
2.5 ml/½ tsp Chinese five-spice powder
45 ml/3 tbsp soy sauce
30 ml/2 tbsp water
225 g/8 oz Chinese egg noodles

1 Separate the onion pieces into layers.
2 Heat the oil in a large non-stick frying pan (skillet) or wok. Add the onion and stir-fry for 2 minutes. Add the pork and stir-fry for 3 minutes.
3 Add the pak choi, garlic, water chestnuts, bamboo shoots and five-spice powder. Stir-fry for a further 2–3 minutes until cooked to your liking. Stir in the soy sauce and water.
4 Put the noodles in a large saucepan. Cover with boiling water and leave to stand for 5 minutes, then drain.
5 Spoon the noodles into large warm bowls. Spoon the pork mixture over and serve straight away.

Dieter's Dream Cheese Soufflé

This is as good as any more calorific version and so easy even a novice cook can't go wrong!

Serves 4

A little low-fat spread, for greasing
100 g/4 oz/½ cup low-fat cheese spread
30 ml/2 tbsp skimmed milk
30 ml/2 tbsp plain (all-purpose) flour
1.5 ml/¼ tsp made English mustard
30 ml/2 tbsp freshly grated Parmesan cheese
Salt and freshly ground black pepper
2 eggs, separated

1 Grease a 15 cm/6 in soufflé dish.
2 Put all the ingredients except the egg whites in a bowl and mix with a wooden spoon until smooth.
3 Whisk the egg whites until stiff and fold in with a metal spoon.
4 Turn the mixture into the soufflé dish and bake in a preheated oven at 190°C/375°F/gas mark 5 (fan oven 170°C) for about 25 minutes until well risen, golden and just set. Serve straight away.

Cauliflower Cheese with Tomatoes
Broccoli is delicious served this way, too.
Serves 4

1 cauliflower, cut into small florets
400 g/14 oz/1 large can of chopped tomatoes
2.5 ml/½ tsp dried mixed herbs
15 g/½ oz/2 tbsp cornflour (cornstarch)
300 ml/½ pt/1¼ cups skimmed milk
A small knob of low-fat spread
Salt and white pepper
75 g/3 oz/¾ cup low-fat Cheddar cheese, grated
5 ml/1 tsp made English mustard
A pinch of cayenne
30 ml/2 tbsp corn flakes, crushed
2 tomatoes, sliced

1 Cook the cauliflower florets in boiling, lightly salted water for about 7 minutes until just tender. Drain and place half in a flameproof dish. Spoon the tomatoes over, sprinkle with the herbs, then top with the remaining cauliflower.
2 Meanwhile, blend the cornflour with a little of the milk in a saucepan. Add the remaining milk and the low-fat spread. Bring to the boil and cook for 1 minute, stirring all the time. Season to taste and stir in 50 g/2 oz/½ cup of the cheese, the mustard and cayenne.

3 Pour the sauce over the cauliflower and sprinkle with the corn flakes and the remaining cheese. Arrange the sliced tomatoes round the edge and heat under a preheated grill (broiler) until golden and bubbling.

Quiche Lorraine

*This is delicious served either warm or cold. For a change, use
100 g/4 oz sliced mushrooms instead of the bacon and sprinkle
with 2.5 ml/½ tsp dried oregano before adding the egg mixture.*

Serves 4

100 g/4 oz/1 cup plain (all-purpose) flour
A pinch of salt
50 g/2 oz/¼ cup low-fat spread
About 30 ml/2 tbsp cold water
2 rashers (slices) of lean streaky bacon, rinded and diced
1 onion, finely chopped
1 egg
200 ml/7 fl oz/scant 1 cup skimmed milk
15 ml/1 tbsp freshly grated Parmesan cheese
Salt and freshly ground black pepper

1 Sift the flour and salt into a bowl. Add the spread and work in
   with a fork until crumbly. Mix with enough of the cold water
   to form a soft but not sticky dough. Wrap in clingfilm (plastic
   wrap) and chill for 30 minutes.
2 Roll out thinly and use to line a 20 cm/8 in flan dish (pie pan).
   Return to the fridge to chill while you prepare the filling.
3 Dry-fry the bacon and onion gently in a frying pan (skillet)
   until the onion has softened and the bacon is cooked but not
   browned. Drain on kitchen paper (paper towels), then tip into
   the flan case (pie shell) and place it on a baking (cookie) sheet.

4 Whisk the egg and milk with the cheese and some salt and pepper. Pour over the bacon and onions.

5 Bake in a preheated oven at 190°C/375°F/gas mark 5 (fan oven 170°C) for about 30 minutes until set and golden brown.

Exotic Mushroom Risotto

If you don't like garlic, simply leave it out – this risotto has lots delicious flavour without it. Supermarkets now sell packets of mixed mushrooms, including shiitake, chestnut, oyster and chanterelles, which are perfect for this recipe but you can use ordinary cup mushrooms for a more economical dish.

Serves 4

15 g/½ oz/1 tbsp low-fat spread
1 onion, finely chopped
1 garlic clove, crushed
225 g/8 oz mixed exotic mushrooms, sliced
225 g/8 oz/1 cup risotto rice
750 ml/1¼ pts/3 cups hot chicken or vegetable stock, made with 2 stock cubes
30 ml/2 tbsp chopped fresh thyme or parsley
Salt and freshly ground black pepper

1 Melt the low-fat spread in a large non-stick saucepan. Add the onion and garlic and fry (sauté), stirring, for 2 minutes until softened but not browned.
2 Add the mushrooms and cook gently for 1 minute, stirring.
3 Stir in the rice and continue to cook gently, stirring, for 1 minute.

4 Add about a quarter of the stock and bring to the boil, stirring. Reduce the heat and simmer gently until the stock is absorbed, stirring occasionally. Repeat, adding a little more stock at a time, until all the stock is used. The rice should be just tender but still with some 'bite' and the mixture should be creamy.

5 Stir in the thyme or parsley and season to taste. Serve straight away.

Pizza Marguerita

*Add a few sliced mushrooms and chopped or sliced (bell)
peppers, if you like, before adding the cheese.*

Serves 4

225 g/8 oz/2 cups plain (all-purpose) flour
10 ml/2 tsp easy-blend dried yeast
5 ml/1 tsp salt
About 150 ml/¼ pt/⅔ cup hand-hot water
45 ml/3 tbsp tomato purée (paste)
15 ml/1 tbsp cold water
Freshly ground black pepper
2.5 ml/½ tsp dried oregano
100 g/4 oz/1 cup low-fat Mozzarella cheese, grated
1 tomato, sliced
1 black olive
A few fresh basil leaves, torn

1 Mix the flour, yeast and salt in a bowl. Mix with enough of
  the hand-hot water to form a soft but not sticky dough. Knead
  for about 3 minutes on a lightly floured surface until smooth
  and elastic.
2 Return to the bowl. Cover the bowl with a damp cloth and
  leave in a warm place for about 45 minutes until doubled in
  bulk.

3 Knock back (punch down) the dough and knead again lightly. Roll out to a large round, about 23 cm/9 in in diameter. Place on a non-stick baking (cookie) sheet.

4 Mix the tomato purée with the cold water and spread out almost to the edges of the dough. Sprinkle with pepper and the oregano.

5 Bake in a preheated oven at 220°C/425°F/gas mark 7 (fan oven 200°C) for 10 minutes. Cover with the cheese, arrange the slices of tomato around and put the olive in the centre.

6 Return to the oven and bake for a further 10 minutes until the dough is crisp and golden and the cheese has melted and is turning lightly brown in places. Sprinkle with the basil and serve straight away.

Desserts

All of the desserts in this section have fewer than 100 calories per portion so, when maintaining the new you, they are ideal for rounding off main meals as a treat. If you feel like indulging yourself even more, turn to pages 184–88, for my desserts for special occasions.

Peach and Orange Fool

You can ring the changes by using canned apricots or pears instead but make sure they are in natural juice, not syrup. Keep the juice to make a fruit salad the following day – simply cut up a selection of fresh fruits and add to the juice.

Serves 4

1 quantity of Velvety Sweet White Sauce (see page 156)
410 g/14½ oz/1 large can of peach slices in natural juice
Grated rind and juice of 1 small orange

1 Make up the sauce and leave to cool.
2 Drain the fruit, reserving the juice. Chop one of the peach slices and set aside for decoration.
3 Purée the remaining fruit with the orange juice in a blender or food processor. Fold in to the sauce with the orange rind.
4 Spoon into glasses and top each with a little of the reserved chopped peach. Chill before serving if time allows.

Strawberry Fluff

Use raspberries and raspberry yoghurt for an equally delicious alternative dessert.

Serves 4

225 g/8 oz ripe strawberries
2 egg whites
300 ml/½ pt/1¼ cups low-calorie strawberry yoghurt

1 Slice the strawberries. Reserve four of the slices for decoration and lightly crush the remainder.
2 Whisk the egg whites until stiff. Fold into the yoghurt.
3 Layer the crushed fruit and fluffy yoghurt in tall glasses and decorate with the reserved fruit.
4 Chill before serving.

Lemon Cream

You can make an orange cream, using an orange instead of the lemon and pure orange juice instead of pineapple. Taste the mixture and, if necessary, add a squeeze of lemon juice to sharpen it.

Serves 4

1 small lemon
10 ml/2 tsp powdered gelatine
300 ml/½ pt/1¼ cups pure pineapple juice
150 ml/¼ pt/⅔ cup low-fat whipping cream, whipped

1 Thinly pare half the rind off the lemon. Cut into thin strips and boil in water for 3 minutes. Drain, rinse with cold water, drain again and set aside for decoration. Finely grate the remaining rind and squeeze the juice.
2 Dissolve the gelatine in a little of the pineapple juice according to the gelatine packet directions. Stir in the remaining pineapple juice.
3 Add the grated lemon rind and as much of the lemon juice as you like to give a good lemony flavour – don't make it too sour.
4 Chill until the consistency of egg white.
5 Gradually whisk into the whipped cream. Transfer to four small dishes and chill until set.
6 Decorate with the reserved thin strips of lemon rind.

Chocolate Hazelnut Mousse

*This dessert is elegant enough for a dinner party too. Use a plain
dark (semi-sweet) chocolate spread, if you prefer.
Rum makes a good substitute for brandy.*

Serves 4

150 ml/¼ pt/⅔ cup low-fat whipping cream
30 ml/2 tbsp chocolate and hazelnut (filbert) spread
15 ml/1 tbsp brandy
A little ground cinnamon

1 Whip the cream until peaking and reserve 30 ml/2 tbsp for
  decoration.
2 Fold the chocolate spread and brandy into the remaining
  cream.
3 Spoon into four demitasse coffee cups or small ramekins
  (custard cups), top with the reserved cream and sprinkle with
  cinnamon. Chill until set.
4 Serve on the coffee saucers if using the cups.

Apple and Banana Flip

*Pears taste good in this instead of apples. I usually flavour them
with cinnamon instead of cloves.*

Serves 4

450 g/1 lb eating (dessert) apples, peeled, cored and sliced
A pinch of ground cloves
45 ml/3 tbsp water
2 ripe bananas, cut into chunks
300 ml/½ pt/1¼ cups low-fat plain yoghurt
8 small angelica 'leaves'

1 Put the apples, cloves and water in a saucepan and stew gently
   until the apples are tender.
2 Cool slightly, then place in a blender with the bananas. Run
   the machine until the mixture is smooth.
3 Leave until completely cold, then gently fold in the yoghurt,
   to give a marbled effect.
4 Spoon into glass dishes and chill.
5 Decorate each with two angelica 'leaves' before serving.

Tangy Orange Mousse

The can of milk must be chilled for several hours beforehand or it will not become foamy when whisked.

Serves 4

1 packet of sugar-free orange jelly (jello) crystals
150 ml/¼ pt/⅔ cup boiling water
300 g/11 oz/1 small can of mandarin oranges in natural juice,
    drained, reserving the juice
15 ml/1 tbsp lemon juice
170 g/6 oz/1 small can of light evaporated milk, chilled
60 ml/4 tbsp low-fat crème fraîche

1 Dissolve the jelly crystals in the boiling water.
2 Stir in the mandarin orange juice and the lemon juice and leave until it has cooled and set to the consistency of egg white.
3 Meanwhile, whisk the evaporated milk until thick and fluffy and fold into the jelly mixture. Reserve four of the mandarin orange segments for decoration and fold the rest into the jelly.
4 Spoon the mousse into glasses and chill until set. Spread the crème fraîche over and decorate with the reserved mandarin orange segments.

Sauces and Dressings

When you are watching your weight, it may seem like a good idea to cut out all dressings, sauces and condiments. However, without them, food can become very dull, with the result that you give up the diet and start piling on the pounds again.

With this in mind, I've put together a selection of sauces and dressings that you can use to add interest and flavour to plain grilled meats or fish, or dress up your healthy salads – without adding too many calories to your meals.

Easy Low-fat White Sauce

You can omit the bouquet garni, if you wish.

Serves 4

20 g/¾ oz/3 tbsp plain (all-purpose) flour
300 ml/½ pt/1¼ cups skimmed milk
A small knob of low-fat spread
1 bouquet garni sachet
A pinch of salt
Freshly ground black or white pepper

1 Put the flour in a saucepan and gradually whisk in the milk.
2 Add the spread and bouquet garni sachet. Bring to the boil and cook for 2 minutes, stirring all the time until thickened and smooth.
3 Squeeze the bouquet garni sachet against the side of the pan to extract the maximum flavour, then discard. Season the sauce to taste with salt and pepper. Use as required.

Variations

Parsley Sauce
Prepare the Easy Low-fat White Sauce, adding add 30 ml/2 tbsp fresh chopped parsley with the seasoning at Step 3.

Cheese Sauce
Prepare the Easy Low-fat White Sauce. Add 50 g/2 oz/½ cup low-fat Cheddar cheese to the cooked sauce and stir until melted.

Mushroom Sauce
Thinly slice or chop 50 g/2 oz button mushrooms. Stew in 30 ml/2 tbsp water in a saucepan until softened. Add the flour and continue from Step 1 as for Easy Low-fat White Sauce.

Velvety Sweet White Sauce

You can make a sweet white sauce with plain (all-purpose) flour but I prefer to use cornflour (cornstarch) as it gives a smoother texture.

Serves 4

15 ml/1 tbsp cornflour
300 ml/½ pt/1¼ cups skimmed milk
15 ml/1 tbsp caster (superfine) sugar
A few drops of vanilla essence (extract)

1 Blend the cornflour with a little of the milk in a saucepan.
2 Add the remaining milk and the sugar.
3 Bring to the boil and cook for 2 minutes until thickened.
4 Stir in the vanilla and use as required.

Variations

Custard Sauce

Prepare as for Velvety Sweet White Sauce, adding a few drops of yellow colouring to the sauce.

Almond Sauce

Prepare as for Velvety Sweet White Sauce but substitute a few drops of almond essence (extract) for the vanilla.

Coffee Sauce

Prepare as for Velvety Sweet White Sauce but blend 5 ml/1 tsp instant coffee with the cornflour before adding the milk.

Chocolate Sauce

Prepare as for Velvety Sweet White Sauce but add 10 ml/2 tsp of cocoa (unsweetened chocolate) powder to the cornflour before blending in the milk. The sauce will be slightly thicker, so thin with 15 ml/1 tbsp skimmed milk, if liked.

Raspberry Sauce

*This is a delicious refreshing sauce, which makes a perfect
dessert partnered with a scoop or two of low-calorie vanilla ice
cream. Alternatively, try it with fresh, sliced tropical fruits, such
as peaches, mangoes, pawpaw and kiwi fruit.*

Serves 4

300 g/11 oz/1 small can of raspberries in natural juice
5 ml/1 tsp clear honey

1 Purée the can of fruit with its juice in a blender or food
   processor, then pass through a sieve (strainer) to remove the
   seeds.
2 Sweeten with the honey.

Virtually Fat-free Vinaigrette Dressing

Salads form an important part of any diet, whether you're watching your weight or not. This dressing is great for adding a zip with just the minimum of calories! Ring the changes using English or grainy mustard instead of Dijon, and other herbs, such as chives or oregano, instead of the tarragon. When you've reached your target weight and are on the maintenance diet, you can add 15 ml/1 tbsp olive oil to the mixture.

Serves 4

30 ml/2 tbsp white wine vinegar
15 ml/1 tbsp water
2.5 ml/½ tsp Dijon mustard
5 ml/1 tsp chopped fresh parsley
5 ml/1 tsp chopped fresh tarragon
A pinch of caster (superfine) sugar
Salt and freshly ground black pepper

1 Whisk the wine vinegar, water and mustard together.
2 Stir in the herbs, sugar and salt and pepper to taste. Use as required.

Chive and Vinegar Dressing
You can use finely chopped spring onions (scallions) instead of chives for an equally delicious dressing.

Serves 4

45 ml/3 tbsp white wine vinegar
15 ml/1 tbsp water
15 ml/1 tbsp Worcestershire sauce
30 ml/2 tbsp snipped fresh chives
Freshly ground black pepper

Mix all the ingredients together and chill before using.

Soy Dressing
This is also delicious with a spoonful or two of very finely chopped cucumber added at the last minute before serving.

Serves 4

30 ml/2 tbsp soy sauce
15 ml/1 tbsp medium-dry sherry
30 ml/2 tbsp water
Salt and freshly ground black pepper

Whisk all the ingredients together and use as required.

Thai Dressing
For a stronger flavour, substitute 5 ml/1 tsp of the soy sauce with Thai fish sauce.

Serves 4

30 ml/2 tbsp soy sauce
5 ml/1 tsp clear honey
1 stem of lemon grass, finely chopped
½ small garlic clove, crushed
Finely grated rind and juice of ½ lime
30 ml/2 tbsp water
Salt and freshly ground black pepper

Put the ingredients in a screw-topped jar. Shake vigorously, then chill for at least 2 hours before using.

Sweet and Sour Dressing
Serves 4

60 ml/4 tbsp pure pineapple juice
5 ml/1 tsp soy sauce
10 ml/2 tsp lemon juice
2.5 ml/½ tsp tomato ketchup (catsup)
Freshly ground black pepper
15 ml/1 tbsp water

Whisk all the ingredients together and use as required.

Tarragon Dressing

You can make other fragrant herb dressings, using fresh, chopped rosemary, basil or chervil instead of the tarragon.

Serves 4

60 ml/4 tbsp white wine vinegar
30 ml/2 tbsp chopped fresh tarragon
A pinch of caster (superfine) sugar
2.5 ml/½ tsp Dijon mustard
30 ml/2 tbsp apple juice
Salt and freshly ground black pepper

1 Put the vinegar in a screw-topped jar with the tarragon, sugar, mustard and apple juice. Season to taste.
2 Shake well and leave to stand for at least 1 hour. Shake again before serving.

Chilli Garlic Dressing

It is important to let this dressing stand for quite a while before use or the flavour will be very mild. If you are in a hurry, chop the seeded chilli and rosemary and crush the garlic, mix the dressing, shake and use immediately.

Serves 4

45 ml/3 tbsp balsamic vinegar
30 ml/2 tbsp cider vinegar
1 fresh red chilli
Salt and freshly ground black pepper
½ garlic clove
1 small sprig of fresh rosemary
30 ml/2 tbsp water

1 Put all the ingredients in a screw-topped jar.
2 Shake vigorously and leave to infuse for several days to allow the flavours to develop. Strain the dressing before using.

Chapter 10
Special-occasion Diet Plan Recipes

Just because you're following a diet plan doesn't have to mean you can't entertain friends for lunch or supper. With the selection of starters, main courses and desserts in this chapter, you can impress your friends and still keep up your diet.

Don't forget that you must eat the meals for the rest of the day from my diet plan for special-occasion days (see page 96). To add to your enjoyment, you can save up your snack allowance for a few extra glasses of wine or a high-calorie dessert instead of choosing one from this section.

I have included suggestions for accompaniments, to provide you – and your guests – with a meal that is nutritionally balanced **and** calorie-wise.

Starters

Dishes for your dinner party or special occasion don't have to be rich in fat and calories. It's far more important that the ingredients are top quality, well prepared and beautifully presented. In fact, the current food trends encourage us to favour simple, light and colourful starters that complement the main meal to follow.

Don't forget – you can also choose one of the soups from the section on pages 104–9. The cold ones are particularly good for a summer lunch or dinner party.

Artichokes with Lemon and Garlic Dressing

You can also serve asparagus with this dressing.

Serves 6

6 globe artichokes
Finely grated rind and juice of ½ lemon
100 g/4 oz/½ cup low-fat spread
1 large garlic clove, crushed
30 ml/2 tbsp chopped fresh parsley
Salt and freshly ground black pepper

1 Twist the stalks off the artichokes and trim off the points of the leaves with scissors, if liked.
2 Add the lemon juice to a pan of boiling, lightly salted water, then drop in the artichokes and cook for about 20 minutes or until a leaf can be pulled off easily. Drain thoroughly and dry upside-down on kitchen paper (paper towels).
3 Meanwhile, put the lemon rind, low-fat spread, garlic and parsley in a saucepan and heat gently. Season to taste with salt and pepper.
4 Spoon the melted mixture into six tiny dishes and place on plates with the artichokes.
5 To eat, pull off the leaves one at a time, dip the fleshy part in the dressing and draw this through the teeth, then discard. When all the leaves are eaten, pull off the small inner leaves at the top and cut away the hairy 'choke'. Eat the base with a knife and fork, dipping it in the remaining dressing.

Sizzled Vine Tomatoes with Mozzarella

If you are still trying to lose weight, have only one thin slice of ciabatta bread and no butter!

Serves 6

30 ml/2 tbsp olive oil
6 small sprigs of vine cherry tomatoes, with 5 or 6 tomatoes on each
10 ml/2 tsp caster (superfine) sugar
30 ml/2 tbsp balsamic vinegar
Salt and freshly ground black pepper
175 g/6 oz reduced-fat Mozzarella cheese, sliced
A handful of fresh basil leaves, torn
Ciabatta bread

1 Heat the oil in a large frying pan (skillet).
2 Add the tomatoes and sprinkle with the sugar. Fry (sauté) for 2 minutes, then carefully turn the sprigs over.
3 Sprinkle with the balsamic vinegar and some salt and pepper. Cover and cook for a further 2–3 minutes until lightly coloured and almost tender but still holding their shape.
4 Arrange the slices of Mozzarella attractively at the side of individual serving plates. Transfer a sprig of tomatoes to each plate and spoon any juices over. Garnish with a few torn basil leaves and serve with ciabatta bread.

Roasted Mediterranean Vegetables with Rosemary and Parma Ham

For a vegetarian version, simply omit the ham and serve with a few sliced black olives scattered over the top.

Serves 6

1 red (bell) pepper, cut into 6 chunky slices
1 green pepper, cut into 6 chunky slices
1 aubergine (eggplant), sliced
1 courgette (zucchini), sliced diagonally
30 ml/2 tbsp olive oil
1 garlic clove, finely chopped
10 ml/2 tsp finely chopped fresh rosemary
Coarse sea salt
6 thin slices of Parma ham
6 small sprigs of fresh rosemary

1 Toss the peppers, aubergine and courgette slices in the oil, garlic and rosemary.
2 Spread them out in a large roasting tin (pan).
3 Roast towards the top of a preheated oven at 200°C/400°F/ gas mark 6 (fan oven 180°C) for 30–40 minutes until tender and lightly charred in places, turning once after 15 minutes.
4 Spoon on to warm plates and sprinkle with a little coarse sea salt. Lay a slice of Parma ham attractively on each plate and serve, garnished with the fresh rosemary.

Pan-grilled Tiger Prawns
with Rocket and Orange Salad
*Grapefruit and lamb's tongue lettuce make a delicious
alternative to the rocket and orange salad.*

Serves 6

50 g/2 oz rocket leaves
2 oranges
1 red onion, thinly sliced
30 ml/2 tbsp balsamic vinegar
Freshly ground black pepper
15 ml/1 tbsp olive oil
36 raw peeled tiger prawns (jumbo shrimp), tails left on

1 Divide the rocket between six plates.
2 Hold the oranges over a bowl and cut off all the rind and pith.
  Slice the fruit into segments, cutting either side of each
  membrane, and scatter the segments over the rocket. Squeeze
  the membranes over the bowl to extract any remaining juice,
  then discard.
3 Separate the onion into rings and scatter over.
4 Whisk the vinegar into the orange juice with a little pepper.
  Sprinkle over the salads.
5 Heat the oil in a large frying pan (skillet) until searingly hot.
  Add the prawns and cook quickly on both sides until just
  turned pink.
6 Arrange on the salads and serve.

Chestnut Mushroom Celery and Carrot Pâté

If you're dieting, have no more than two triangles of toast.

Serves 6

40 g/1½ oz/3 tbsp low-fat spread
1 onion, finely chopped
2 celery sticks, grated, discarding any strings
2 carrots, grated
350 g/12 oz chestnut mushrooms, finely chopped
15 ml/1 tbsp lemon juice
200 g/7 oz/1 small carton of low-fat soft cheese
30 ml/2 tbsp fresh chopped parsley
Salt and freshly ground black pepper
A few sprigs of fresh parsley
Triangles of hot toast

1 Melt the spread in a saucepan. Add the onion, celery and carrot and cook, stirring, for 2 minutes until softened.
2 Add the mushrooms and lemon juice, then cover and cook gently, stirring occasionally, for 5 minutes until tender and no liquid remains. If necessary, boil rapidly to evaporate any remaining liquid. Turn into a bowl to cool.
3 Beat in the cheese, parsley and salt and pepper to taste. Spoon into small pots and level the surfaces. Chill until ready to serve.
4 Garnish each pot with a sprig of parsley and serve with triangles of hot toast.

Oriental Vegetable Soup

If you are dieting, don't have more than four prawn crackers.

Serves 6

15 ml/1 tbsp sunflower oil
1 small garlic clove, crushed
3 spring onions (scallions), diagonally sliced
50 g/2 oz very thin French (green) beans, trimmed and cut into
    short lengths
4 baby corn cobs, cut into 1 cm/½ in chunks
50 g/2 oz shiitake or button mushrooms, thinly sliced
1 carrot, cut into tiny matchsticks
1 small red (bell) pepper, cut into tiny matchsticks
1 small green chilli, seeded and thinly sliced
900 ml/1½ pts/3¾ cups vegetable or chicken stock, made with
    2 stock cubes
15 ml/1 tbsp soy sauce
15 ml/1 tbsp oyster sauce
15 ml/1 tbsp medium-dry sherry
Prawn crackers, to serve

1 Heat the oil in a large saucepan and stir-fry the garlic and
   prepared vegetables for 3 minutes until glistening in the oil.
2 Add the stock, soy sauce, oyster sauce and sherry. Bring to the
   boil, reduce the heat and simmer for 5 minutes until the
   vegetables are just tender but still have some 'bite'.
3 Ladle into warm bowls and serve with prawn crackers.

Main Courses

There are dishes here to suit all occasions – lunches, informal suppers and more formal dinners. Don't forget the importance of presentation when you are preparing a special-occasion meal. Think about the colour and texture of the main course and side dishes you choose, and choose combinations that add contrast as well as complementing each other. To set off the food to perfection, add a little garnish before serving – just a sprinkling of chopped fresh herbs, a slice of lemon or a dusting of bright red paprika will do wonders.

Beef Shiraz

Don't be tempted to put any butter on your jacket potato!
If you are vegetarian, make this with reconstituted soya protein
or Quorn chunks.

Serves 6

700 g/1½ lb lean braising steak, diced
30 ml/2 tbsp plain (all-purpose) flour
Salt and freshly ground black pepper
50 g/2 oz lean bacon, finely diced
1 garlic clove, crushed
350 g/12 oz button (pearl) onions
225 g/8 oz small button mushrooms, wiped
2 carrots, sliced

2 turnips, quartered and sliced
450 ml/³/₄ pt/2 cups Shiraz red wine
200 ml/7 fl oz/scant 1 cup beef stock, made with 1 stock cube
15 ml/1 tbsp tomato purée (paste)
1 bouquet garni sachet
Snipped fresh chives, for garnishing
Jacket-baked potatoes and broccoli, to serve

1 Toss the meat in the flour with a little salt and pepper added. Place in a large flameproof casserole dish (Dutch oven) with all the remaining ingredients.
2 Bring to the boil, stirring gently. Cover with the lid and transfer to a preheated oven at 160°C/325°F/gas mark 3 (fan oven 140°C). Cook for 2½–3 hours until the meat is really tender.
3 Stir well, remove the bouquet garni, taste and add more salt and pepper if necessary.
4 Sprinkle the casserole with the chives and serve with jacket-baked potatoes and broccoli.

Swiss Fondue Chicken Pies

For vegetarians, use Quorn steaks or nut cutlets instead of the chicken.

Serves 6

1 garlic clove, halved
200 ml/7 fl oz/scant 1 cup chicken stock, made with ½ stock cube
75 ml/5 tbsp dry white wine
6 skinless chicken breasts
Salt and freshly ground black pepper
6 sheets of filo pastry (paste)
15 g/½ oz/1 tbsp low-fat spread, melted
450 g/1 lb baby spinach leaves
A good pinch of grated nutmeg
5 ml/1 tsp cornflour (cornstarch)
15 ml/1 tbsp water
100 g/4 oz/1 cup reduced-fat Cheddar cheese, grated
75 ml/5 tbsp low-fat crème fraîche
30 ml/2 tbsp chopped fresh parsley
Baby carrots and mangetout (snow peas), to serve

1 Rub the garlic clove round the base of a large saucepan and discard.
2 Put the stock and wine in the pan and add the chicken and a little salt and pepper. Bring to the boil, then reduce the heat, cover and cook gently for 10 minutes until cooked through.

3 Carefully lift the chicken out of the pan, wrap in foil and keep warm.

4 Meanwhile, brush each pastry sheet with a little of the melted spread. Scrunch each sheet gently so that it looks like crumpled paper and place on a non-stick baking (cookie) sheet. Bake in a preheated oven at 190°C/375°F/gas mark 5 (fan oven 170°C) for about 8–10 minutes until golden.

5 While the pastry and chicken cook, wash the spinach well, then shake to remove excess water and place in a saucepan. Sprinkle with pepper and nutmeg. Cover and cook gently for just 3 minutes until wilted but not mushy. Drain in a colander.

6 When the chicken is cooked, boil the cooking liquid rapidly for 3 minutes until reduced by half. Blend the cornflour with the water and stir into the liquid until thickened and clear. Add the cheese and crème fraîche and stir until completely melted, thick and smooth.

7 Cut the chicken diagonally into slices. Spoon the spinach into the centres of six warm plates. Arrange the chicken on top, then spoon a little of the cheese fondue mixture over.

8 Top each with a piece of baked crumpled filo pastry and scatter the parsley over. Serve hot with baby carrots and mangetout.

Spiced Lamb with Apricots and Couscous

*For a meatless version, use three 425 g/15 oz/large cans of
chickpeas (garbanzos) instead of the lamb.
The recipe also works well with tofu.*

Serves 6

700 g/ 1½ lb lamb neck fillets, cut into chunks
Salt and freshly ground black pepper
2.5 ml/½ tsp ground cumin
2.5 ml/½ tsp ground ginger
5 ml/1 tsp paprika
1 garlic clove, crushed
1 bunch of spring onions (scallions), chopped
1 green (bell) pepper, diced
175 g/6 oz/1 cup ready-to-eat dried apricots, halved
600 ml/1 pt/2½ cups lamb or chicken stock, made with 1 stock
cube
45 ml/3 tbsp tomato purée (paste)
15 ml/1 tbsp clear honey
4 courgettes (zucchini), sliced
350 g/12 oz/3 cups couscous
90 ml/6 tbsp low-fat crème fraîche and a few torn fresh
coriander (cilantro) leaves, for garnishing
A green salad, to serve

1 Mix the lamb with some salt and pepper, the spices, garlic, spring onions, green pepper and apricots in a large flameproof casserole dish (Dutch oven).
2 Add the stock, tomato purée and honey. Bring to the boil, stirring gently, reduce the heat to low, cover and simmer very gently, stirring occasionally for 1 hour.
3 Add the courgettes and continue to simmer, uncovered, for 15 minutes until tender and bathed in a rich sauce.
4 Meanwhile, cook the couscous according to the packet directions and fluff up with a fork.
5 Spoon the couscous on to warm plates and top with the lamb mixture. Add a spoonful of crème fraîche and a few torn coriander leaves. Serve with a green salad.

Lamb Steaks with Mint Jus and Leek Mash

Instead of lamb steaks, you can use lamb neck fillets. You need only 75–100 g/3–4 oz per person. Cut them into slices, place between sheets of clingfilm (plastic wrap), flatten with a meat mallet or rolling pin, and fry (sauté) quickly on both sides until browned and just cooked.

Serves 6

900 g/2 lb potatoes
2 large leeks
2 large carrots
2 courgettes (zucchini)
25 g/1 oz/2 tbsp low-fat spread
6 lamb steaks, trimmed of any fat
Salt and freshly ground black pepper
20 ml/1½ tbsp cornflour (cornstarch)
30 ml/2 tbsp bottled garden mint
5 ml/1 tsp clear honey

1 Peel and cut the potatoes into small, even-sized chunks. Place in a pan of cold, lightly salted water.
2 Trim the leeks, cut almost right through from the green tops to the white root end and wash well under cold, running water. Chop and add to the potatoes.

3 Pare the carrots and courgettes into thin strips with a potato peeler. Place in a colander or steamer over the potato pan. Bring to the boil, reduce the heat, part-cover and simmer for about 8 minutes until all the vegetables are tender. Drain, reserving the cooking liquid. Keep the carrots and courgettes warm.

4 Mash the potatoes and leeks with half the low-fat spread and keep warm.

5 Melt the remaining spread and brush over the lamb steaks on both sides. Season lightly.

6 Place on foil on the grill (broiler) rack and grill (broil) for 5–8 minutes on each side until cooked to your liking. Transfer to a plate and keep warm.

7 Tip the cooking juices on the foil into a small saucepan and scrape any sediment off the foil. Stir in the cornflour and garden mint. Measure 450 ml/¾ pt/2 cups of the potato and leek cooking water and pour into the pan, stirring to blend completely. Add the honey. Bring to the boil, and cook for 1 minute, stirring all the time. Season to taste.

8 Spoon a mound of leek mash on to the centres of six warm plates. Top each with a lamb steak. Spoon the mint jus over and put a small pile of carrot and courgette at the side. Serve straight away.

Thai-style Turkey with Sesame Seeds

*This is just as good made with Quorn or reconstituted
soya pieces for vegetarians.*

Serves 6

700 g/1½ lb turkey breast steaks, cut into short strips
2 red onions, halved and thinly sliced
1 red chilli, seeded and chopped
Finely grated rind and juice of 1 lime
Finely grated rind and juice of ½ lemon
2 garlic cloves, crushed
30 ml/2 tbsp Thai fish sauce
10 ml/2 tsp soft dark brown sugar
1 stalk of lemon grass, finely chopped
5 ml/1 tsp sesame oil
30 ml/2 tbsp sunflower oil
30 ml/2 tbsp sesame seeds
Salt and freshly ground black pepper
350 g/12 oz rice noodles
1 each of red, green and yellow (bell) peppers, cut into very
    fine strips
30 ml/2 tbsp soy sauce
1 small head of Chinese leaves (stem lettuce), shredded
45 ml/3 tbsp balsamic vinegar

1 Put the turkey and onions in a bowl. Add the chilli, lime and lemon rinds and juices, garlic, fish sauce, sugar, lemon grass, sesame oil, half the sunflower oil, the sesame seeds and a little salt and pepper. Stir well and leave to marinate for 2 hours.

2 Cook the rice noodles according to the packet directions. Drain.

3 Cook the pepper strips in boiling water for 4 minutes. Drain and keep warm.

4 Heat the remaining oil in a large wok or frying pan (skillet). Add the turkey mixture and stir-fry for 4–5 minutes until cooked through. Stir in 10 ml/2 tsp of the soy sauce.

5 Put the shredded Chinese leaves in a salad bowl with the balsamic vinegar and the remaining soy sauce. Toss with a little black pepper.

6 Spoon the noodles into warm bowls. Top each with turkey mixture, then a few of the mixed pepper strips. Serve straight away with the Chinese leaf salad.

Gourmet Fish and Chips

Don't use oven chips for this recipe – they are coated in fat! If you like spicy food, add a freshly chopped chilli to the sauce.

Serves 6

6 cod or haddock fillets, about 150 g/5 oz each, skinned
150 g/5 oz/2½ cups fresh breadcrumbs
30 ml/2 tbsp chopped fresh parsley
15 ml/1 tbsp chopped fresh thyme
15 ml/1 tbsp dried onion granules
Salt and freshly ground black pepper
2 egg whites
15 ml/1 tbsp water
700 g/1½ lb frozen chips (fries)
75 ml/5 tbsp low-calorie mayonnaise
75 ml/5 tbsp low-fat crème fraîche
15 ml/1 tbsp capers, chopped
6 gherkins (cornichons), finely chopped
1 canned pimiento cap, drained and finely chopped
A few wedges of lemon and sprigs of watercress, for garnishing
Mangetout and baby carrots, to serve

1 Wipe the fish and remove any remaining bones.
2 Mix the breadcrumbs with half the parsley, the thyme, dried onion granules and some salt and pepper in a shallow dish.

3 Beat the egg whites with the water in a separate dish.

4 Dip the fish in the egg white, then in the breadcrumbs, to coat completely. Place on a non-stick baking (cookie) sheet.

5 Spread out the chips on a separate baking sheet.

6 Place the chips on the top shelf of the oven, preheated to 220°C/425°F/gas mark 7 (fan oven 200°C), with the fish on the shelf below. Cook for 30 minutes until golden and cooked through.

7 Meanwhile, make the sauce. Mix the mayonnaise with the crème fraîche, capers, gherkins and chopped pimiento. Add a good grinding of pepper, then fold in the remaining chopped parsley. Spoon the sauce into a small serving bowl.

8 Transfer the fish and chips to warm plates. Garnish with lemon wedges and sprigs of watercress and serve with the sauce, mangetout and baby carrots.

Desserts

The thing most people look forward to when they go out for a meal is the dessert, but for anyone who's watching their weight that's usually the first thing to be cut out. However, there's no need to deprive yourself – or your guests – if you choose from the selection on the next few pages. These puddings all have around 100 calories and some have even fewer, providing the perfect end to your dinner party.

Zabaglione with Raspberries

Zabaglione can also be served plain, with a single sponge finger (lady finger) tucked down the side.

Serves 6

3 eggs
75 ml/5 tbsp medium-dry sherry
30 ml/2 tbsp caster (superfine) sugar
175 g/6 oz fresh or thawed frozen raspberries

1 Put the eggs, sherry and caster sugar in a large bowl over a pan of gently simmering water.
2 Whisk with an electric beater until thick, pale and foamy.
3 Spoon the raspberries into wine glasses and spoon the egg mixture on top. Serve straight away.

Grilled Spiced Pineapple

This is very simple to make but the green tops give it a very special, exotic look. If you can't get baby pineapples, use a large one, cut into six wedges.

Serves 6

3 baby pineapples
60 ml/4 tbsp clear honey
10 ml/2 tsp ground cinnamon
120 ml/4 fl oz/½ cup low-fat crème fraîche

1 Quarter the pineapples lengthways, leaving the green stalks on. Wrap the green parts in foil to protect them.
2 Mix half the honey with the cinnamon. Lay a sheet of foil on the grill (broiler) rack and lay the pineapple pieces on this, skin-sides down. Brush all over the flesh with the mixture.
3 Cook under the preheated grill for about 5 minutes until lightly caramelised, turning the fruit if necessary.
4 Transfer to plates and remove the foil round the green tops.
5 Put a spoonful of crème fraîche to one side and drizzle a little of the remaining honey over the top. Serve warm.

Rhubarb and Orange Meringue Cups
Serves 6

450 g/1 lb rhubarb, cut into 2.5 cm/1 in lengths
A good pinch of bicarbonate of soda (baking soda)
100 g/4 oz/½ cup caster (superfine) sugar
6 oranges
2 egg whites

1 Put the rhubarb in a saucepan with the bicarbonate of soda and 25 g/1 oz/2 tbsp of the sugar.
2 Finely grate the rind from the bottom (not the stalk end) of each orange into the rhubarb, then cut off the grated piece, revealing the fruit inside. Scoop the fruit out with a spoon, chop and add to the rhubarb. Reserve the orange shells.
3 Heat the rhubarb fairly gently until the juice runs, then cover with a lid and cook for about 10 minutes, stirring occasionally until pulpy.
4 Put the orange shells in six individual ovenproof dishes. Spoon the rhubarb mixture inside.
5 Whisk the egg whites until stiff. Gradually whisk in half the remaining sugar until stiff again, then fold in the remainder with a metal spoon. Spoon on top of the oranges.
6 Bake in a preheated oven at 230°C/450°F/gas mark 8 (fan oven 210°C) for 2–3 minutes until the peaks are just turning golden.
7 Serve straight away.

Minted Blackcurrant Frost
Try this with raspberries and raspberry cordial too.

Serves 6

450 g/1 lb blackcurrants
75 g/3 oz/⅓ cup caster (superfine) sugar
30 ml/2 tbsp finely chopped fresh mint
30 ml/2 tbsp sugar-free blackcurrant cordial
150 ml/¼ pt/⅔ cup red wine
A few small sprigs of fresh mint, for garnishing

1 Select six small sprigs of blackcurrants and reserve for decoration. Remove the remainder from their stalks, using the prongs of a fork, and place in a saucepan.
2 Add the sugar, mint, cordial and wine. Bring slowly to the boil, then reduce the heat and stew for 5 minutes until soft.
3 Cool slightly, then purée roughly in a blender or food processor. Don't make it completely smooth – you want some texture to the finished dish.
4 Tip the mixture into a freezer-proof container and leave until completely cold. Freeze for 2 hours, then tip into a bowl and whisk with a fork to break up the ice crystals. Freeze again until just firm.
5 Transfer to the fridge 15 minutes before you wish to serve, to allow it to soften a little.
6 Serve in long-stemmed glasses with a sprig of blackcurrants draped over each glass and add a sprig of mint on top.

Poached Pears with Ice Cream and Chocolate Sauce

You must use drinking (sweetened) chocolate powder with milk powder already added.

Serves 6

3 large pears, peeled, halved and cored
300 ml/½ pt/1¼ cups apple juice
1 piece of cinnamon stick
100 g/4 oz/1 cup instant low-calorie drinking chocolate powder
A little boiling water
6 scoops of low-calorie vanilla ice cream
15 ml/1 tbsp toasted chopped mixed nuts

1 Place the pears in a saucepan with the apple juice and cinnamon. Bring to the boil, reduce the heat, cover and simmer for 5 minutes.
2 Carefully turn the pears over and cook for a further 5 minutes or until just tender but still holding their shape. Do not overcook or they will go mushy. Leave to cool in the liquid.
3 When nearly ready to serve, using a wire whisk, mix the chocolate powder with boiling water, a spoonful at a time, until the mixture forms a thick, smooth pouring sauce.
4 Drain the pear halves and place, cut side up, in individual glass dishes. Put a scoop of ice cream on top. Spoon a little chocolate sauce over, sprinkle with nuts and serve straight away.

Index

alcohol 27, 46
  snack allowances 58, 60, 61
appetite suppressants 22–23
apple and banana flip 152
artichokes with lemon and garlic
  dressing 166
aubergines
  mixed moussaka 116–117

bacon
  spaghetti carbonara 127
beef
  beef chow mein 112
  beef shiraz 172–173
beef, minced
  chilli con carne 120
  cottage pie 124–125
  lasagne 118–119
beetroot soup, Russian 109
biscuits 47, 53
  snack allowances 58, 59, 60–61
blackcurrant frost, minted 187
body toning diets 12
breakfast 53, 55, 63
  breakfast smoothie 63

caffeine 27
cakes
  snack allowances 58, 59, 60–61
calcium 26
calories
  burnt during activities 38–39
  calorie-counted diets 13
  daily allowance 33
  maintaining weight loss 100–101

carrot and coriander soup 104
cauliflower cheese with tomatoes 140–1
cereals 25
cheese
  cauliflower cheese with
    tomatoes 140–1
  cheesy-topped prawn bake 133
chewing gum 64
chicken
  chicken and vegetable stir-fry 110–111
  chicken fajitas 114–115
  individual chicken and mushroom
    pies 122–123
  sweet and sour chicken 113
  Swiss fondue chicken pies 174–175
chilled cucumber and mint soup 107
chilli con carne 120
chocolate 47
  chocolate hazelnut mousse 151
  snack allowances 57, 59
clubs (slimming) 21
cottage pie 124–125
couscous
  spiced lamb with apricots and
    couscous 176–177
cucumber and mint soup, chilled 107

dairy products 26
desserts
  apple and banana flip 152
  chocolate hazelnut mousse 151
  grilled spiced pineapple 185
  lemon cream 150
  minted blackcurrant frost 187
  peach and orange fool 148

poached pears with ice cream and chocolate sauce 188
rhubarb and orange meringue cups 186
snack allowances 58, 59
strawberry fluff 149
tangy orange mousse 153
zabaglione with raspberries 184
detox diets 14
diet plan (28-day) 65–94
  special occasions 96
dieter's dream cheese soufflé 139
diets 7–9, 11
  body toning 12
  calorie-counted diets 13
  detox diets 14
  exchange plans 15
  fad diets 16
  food-combining diets 17
  high-protein, low-carbohydrate diets 18
  low-fat diets 19
  replacement meal diets 20
  slimming clubs 21
  slimming pills 22–23
diuretics 22–23
dressings
  chilli garlic 163
  chive and vinegar 160
  sweet and sour 161
  tarragon 162
  Thai 161
  virtually fat-free vinaigrette 159

easy low-fat white sauce 154–155
essential fats 26–27
exchange plans 15
exercise 34–39
  non-intrusive 35–37

part of life 37–39
exotic mushroom risotto 144–145

facial toning (exercises) 35
fad diets 16
fajitas, chicken 114–115
fat attackers 22
fats 26–27
  cooking in 31
  cutting down on 48–49
fish
  fish cakes 128–129
  fish pie 130–131
  gourmet fish and chips 182–183
  see also salmon
fluids 27
food-combining diets 17
fruit 25, 50
  snack allowances 62

grains 25

ham
  roasted Mediterranean vegetables with rosemary Parma ham 168
Hay diet 17
healthy eating 24–31
high-protein, low-carbohydrate diets 18
hunger, dealing with 64
  see also snacks; weight loss

ice cream
  snack allowances 58, 59, 61
Irish stew 136

lamb
  Irish stew 136
  lamb steaks with mint jus and leek mash 178–179

spiced lamb with apricots and couscous 176–177
lasagne 118–119
leek and potato soup 105
lemon cream 150
lifestyle quiz 40–54
limbering up 36–37
low-calorie pasta salad 121
low-fat diets 19
low-fat spreads 48

meals, balanced 49–51
men on the diet 55, 66
moussaka, mixed 116–117
Mozzarella cheese
  sizzled vine tomatoes with Mozzarella 167
mushroom risotto, exotic 144–145

noodles
  beef chow mein 112

orange mousse, tangy 153

pasta
  low-calorie pasta salad 121
  tuna, sweetcorn and tomato pasta bake 137
  see also lasagne, spaghetti, tagliatelle
pâtés
  chestnut mushroom celery and carrot pâté 170
peach and orange fool 148
pears
  poached pears with ice cream and chocolate sauce 188
pies
  individual chicken and mushroom pies 122–123

Swiss fondue chicken pies 174–175
pills (slimming) 22–23
pineapple, grilled spiced 185
pizza Marguerita 146–147
pork, bamboo and water chestnut stir-fry with noodles 138
potatoes 25
prawns
  cheesy-topped prawn bake 133
  pan-grilled tiger prawns with rocket and orange salad 169
proteins 26

quiche Lorraine 142–143
quiz, lifestyle 40–54

raspberry sauce 158
replacement meal diets 20
restaurant meals 97–99
rhubarb and orange meringue cups 186
risotto, exotic mushroom 144–145
Russian beetroot soup 109

salad, low-calorie pasta 121
salmon
  salmon parcels 134–135
  smoked salmon and broccoli tagliatelle 132
sauces
  easy low-fat white 154–155
  raspberry 158
  velvety sweet white 156–157
savoury snacks 58, 59, 61
shepherd's pie 124–125
slimming
  clubs 21
  pills 22–23
snacks 50, 56–62
soufflés
  dieter's dream cheese soufflé 139

soup 50–51
  carrot and coriander 104
  chilled cucumber and mint 107
  leek and potato 105
  Oriental vegetable 171
  Russian beetroot 109
  tomato and orange 106–107
  vegetable 108
  see also starters
spaghetti
  carbonara 127
  with tomato and basil sauce 126
special occasions 95–99
starch blockers 22
starchy food 25
starters 165
  artichokes with lemon and garlic
    dressing 166
  chestnut mushroom celery and
    carrot pâté 170
  pan-grilled tiger prawns with rocket
    and orange salad 169
  roasted Mediterranean vegetables
    with rosemary Parma ham 168
  sizzled vine tomatoes with
    Mozzarella 167
  see also soup
stir-fries
  chicken and vegetable stir-fry 110–111
  pork, bamboo and water chestnut
    stir-fry with noodles 138
strawberry fluff 149
sugars 27, 30
sweet and sour
  chicken 113
  dressing 161

sweets 47
  snack allowances 57, 59, 60

tagliatelle
  smoked salmon and broccoli
    tagliatelle 132
tarragon dressing 162
Thai dressing 161
Thai-style turkey with sesame seeds
  180–181
tomato and orange soup 106–107
tuna, sweetcorn and tomato pasta
  bake 137
turkey
  Thai-style turkey with sesame
    seeds 180–181

vegetables 25, 50–51
  Oriental vegetable soup 171
  snack allowances 62
vegetable soup 108
vegetarians 64
velvety sweet white sauce 156–157
virtually fat-free vinaigrette dressing 159

water
  aid to weight loss 29
  in diet 27
weight
  chart 28
  target weight 28–29
weight loss
  and health 32–34
  maintaining 100–101
  making it easier 29–31, 46–54, 64
  plateau effect 33

zabaglione with raspberries 184